Yvonne, I have many great memories of us power walking together - May God continue to bless you and your family always!

Love ya, J Shell

# *Fit For His Service*

## *A Life of Intensity*

AF699202

J. Shell

CROSSBOOKS
PUBLISHING

*CrossBooks™*
*A Division of LifeWay*
*1663 Liberty Drive*
*Bloomington, IN 47403*
*www.crossbooks.com*
*Phone: 1-866-879-0502*

*©2010 J. Shell. All rights reserved.*

*No part of this book may be reproduced, stored in a retrieval system, or transmitted by any means without the written permission of the author.*

*First published by CrossBooks 10/11/2010*

*ISBN: 978-1-6150-7225-5 (sc)*

*Library of Congress Control Number: 2010905768*

Scripture taken from the New King James Version. Copyright 1979, 1980, 1982 by Thomas Nelson, inc. Used by permission. All rights reserved.

Scripture taken from the King James Version of the Bible.

Scripture taken from the HOLY BIBLE, NEW INTERNATIONAL VERSION®. Copyright © 1973, 1978, 1984 Biblica. Used by permission of Zondervan. All rights reserved.

Scripture quotations taken from the New American Standard Bible Copyright © 1960, 1962, 1963, 1968, 1971, 1972, 1973, 1975, 1977, 1995 by The Lockman Foundation Used by permission." (www.Lockman.org)

*Scripture taken from The Message. Copyright ? 1993, 1994, 1995, 1996, 2000, 2001, 2002. Used by permission of NavPress Publishing Group."*

Scripture quotations are taken from the Holy Bible, New Living Translation, copyright 1996, 2004. Used by permission of Tyndale House Publishers, Inc., Wheaton, Illinois 60189. All rights reserved.

*Printed in the United States of America*

*This book is printed on acid-free paper.*

Have you ever been fed physically, emotionally and spiritually all at the same time? Well, that is what Fit For His Service did for me! It helped me sort out why I am overeating and why I did not have the desire to follow through on any program for more than a few weeks! It deals with each aspect of your life and why we do what we do.

The eating program is so simple and it works great if you follow it. June Shell designed this after years of trying and not succeeding. Then God gave her the victory and desire to help other women get out of the rut! The fellowship with the other ladies in the same situation was so comforting and rewarding to me. The desire of every woman is to feel loved and attractive. So, if you are ready to pursue the life long journey of not dieting but a way of life that includes eating right, exercise and journaling as you see results, then this is the study for you.

Sheila Watson
Fit for His Service Class Participant
Harp's Crossing Baptist Church
Fayetteville, Ga.

"Fit for His Service" What a great title! I have spent most of my life unfit and unhealthy and missed so many opportunities when health issues held me back from serving my Savior and living the abundant life. This program is written to help you realize how important you are to God and the great design he has for each life. The Holy Spirit has inspired June to help others through her own weight loss journey. Her commitment to health stems from her love for the Savior and she freely shares her knowledge as a personal trainer with everyone who will listen.

I loved the concept of the "Circle of Health" because I am such an "all or nothing" person. June helps you understand that even if you can only do one of the five parts of the circle, you are adding to your health. There is freedom to be found in this program.

She teaches you how to love and take care of your mind, body and spirit through the finished work of Christ on the cross and learning how to forgive yourself when you fail. This is far from a fad diet but true wisdom from

God sprinkled with the knowledge of a personal trainer which cultivates a desire to do better in every area of your life. You will truly be changed inside and out through "Fit for His Service."

Debbie Grulke "a work in progress"
Fit for His Service Class Participant
Harp's Crossing Baptist Church
Fayetteville, Ga.

# Acknowledgements

1 Corinthians 15:57...All praise be to God who gives us the victory through our Lord Jesus Christ!

I am continuously surprised that God allows me to be used by Him. The greatest joy of my life has been in serving Him. God has never allowed me to go through anything that He hasn't later used to allow me to help someone else. That is what this book is all about.
When God first began to speak to my heart concerning the writing of this program, little did I know what blessings were in store for me.

When I walked up to my Pastor's wife at church and told her I was writing a health and fitness study for the ladies of our church, she looked at me and simply said, "Hurry up!" What encouragement!

That was just the beginning!
My daughter Kim was my listening ear for the entire first year of my writing. She allowed me to bounce every idea for the class and program off of her. Her selfless gift of time and encouragement during this process has been priceless to me.

My son Stephen was also a huge part of this process working with me to format the concept of the Circle of Health.

My daughter-in-law Erin, who said to me one day during the first class, "Hey, tell your ladies something I read today, to fast on things of the world and feast on things of God!" Your interest has been great encouragement to me!

My Mother who is turning 81 this month and still power walks in the mornings; you are my inspiration!

I am grateful to my Pastor and the entire staff at Harp's Crossing Baptist Church for their support and encouragement during this process.

My friends and prayer warriors, Debbie, Angela, Elaine, Sheila...as I write this, my heart overflows with love for you.

My six little reasons for staying fit: Emma, Ella, Anna, Emily, Nathan and Daniel…Nanny loves you all!

I want to thank my best friend and encourager, my husband Mike, who simply believes in me! I love you!

May this book be used to help others to grow closer to the Lord Jesus Christ and for the uplifting of His Kingdom.

*Make a joyful noise unto the Lord, all you lands!*
*Serve the Lord with gladness!*
*Come before His presence with singing.*
*Know that the Lord, He is God.*
*It is He who has made us and not we ourselves.*
*We are His people and the sheep of His pasture.*
*Enter into His gates with thanksgiving, and into His courts with praise!*
*Be thankful to Him and Bless His Name!*
*For the Lord is good!*
*His mercy is everlasting*
*And*
*His truth endures to all generations.*
*Psalm 100*

# Contents

# Introduction

# Welcome to Fit for His Service

- *Anything that causes us to be less than what God created us to be . . .*
- *Is not God's will for our lives . . .*
- *Should not be in our lives . . .*
- *Should not be a part of our lives!*

Dear Sisters in Christ,

After years of struggling with weight issues caused by unhealthy eating and a sedentary lifestyle, God did a mighty work in my life and freed me from the bondage of unhealthy living.

I strongly believe that God wants us to live *A Life of Intensity* for Him. Our daily existence matters to Him. He loves us and wants what is best for each one of us. He came so we could not only have eternal life, but also live an abundant life while we are here.

No matter what your age, current weight, occupation, marital status, etc. God will meet you where you are right now. All you have to do is call on Him. He is waiting for you.

This program is dedicated to my Sisters at Harp's Crossing Baptist Church in Fayetteville, Georgia. However, my heart is for *all* ladies to be set free from the bondage and pain that excess weight and unhealthy living can cause. I pray that each one of you will glean from this program what God has in mind for you individually.

The program works best when done in a group setting with a leader who can help you through the first twelve weeks. Remember, this is just a jump start! The habits you will form during these twelve weeks will be with you for the rest of your life.

If you are unable to attend a group setting at this time, then follow the Circle of Health and you *will* achieve results.

Before you begin this program, your personal state of health should be evaluated. Consult your physician before beginning this journey.

# The Journey Begins!

Congratulations! If you are reading this, you have decided to do something about the condition of your health! I am excited for you because I know that this is no accident. You have been prayed for and considered during the writing of this program. I am also excited because the day you begin this program is the day you will begin to feel better physically, and will also begin to feel better about yourself. You will see many things repeated in this program, mostly to drive home the points…one of the main ones you will see is that God loves us and wants us to be healthy! He wants the very best for each of us in all areas of our lives!

Below is a list of things I will be asking you to do before you begin this program. Many of them will need to be continued and renewed throughout the program.

1. Pray about being on the program. Ask God to help you even before you begin, to have a positive mindset concerning the program.
    - Commit to the program for 12 weeks.
    - Be prepared to attend twelve group sessions.
2. Pray for others that will also be starting the program.
3. Pray for the leaders of the program.
4. Have an up-to-date physical visit with your doctor to get clearance to begin the program. Tell him that you are beginning a program of nutrition and mild to moderate cardiovascular exercise and strength training. Tell him or her that you will be incorporating hydration into your daily life. We are trying to drink about ½ of our current weight in ounces of water each day. This is also individual and needs to be approved by your physician.
5. Get a letter of clearance.
6. Let your close friends and family members know that you are beginning a health and fitness program. Ask them to pray for you and encourage you along the way. Let your family know that things will have to be different in order for you to be

successful. Let them know how important this is to you and ask them to be flexible and encouraging.

7. Begin to assess your kitchen, refrigerator, freezer and pantry. Clear out things that you already know to be unhealthy and lacking nutritional value.
8. Go to the restaurants where you and your family eat. Ask them for a list of nutritional information on their food. For many restaurants this can be obtained online from their websites.
9. You will need a good pair of cross training tennis shoes.
10. You will need some good thick exercise socks.
11. You will need some loose fitting exercise clothes, such as sweat clothes, etc.
12. You will need a large insulated lunch carrier.
13. You will need a large water bottle to carry with you.
14. Last, but not least—this may be difficult—start a journal. Begin with an assessment of your current health. Make a list of the current medicines you are on. Also include on this list over-the-counter items needed, and about how often you take them. Include anything you take: for headaches, other aches and pains, indigestion problems, constipation, etc. Be sure to include health issues such as reflux, arthritis, inability to sleep, etc. How are these affecting you, your life, your family and your area of service? Are you able to do all the things you would like to do? Or are health issues stemming from excess weight or stress holding you back? Instead of being down on yourself when you are writing this, realize that this is the beginning of a totally new way of life. Again, congratulations on a new beginning. Together, with God's help, we will become Fit for His Service!

# Fit for His Service Group Meetings

*This is for those of you who like to know what to expect…

Fit for His Service is designed to be used in a group setting. The following are some of the questions that are frequently asked about the class itself. Your leader or facilitator will tailor this to meet your group's specific needs.

***What will class be like?***

To begin, we will have to do some housekeeping, such as taking a waist measurement on everyone. This will be done in private and will be totally confidential.

Each class will consist of a Bible study. These are based on encouraging scriptures to help us along the way. This will be a time of focusing on Jesus and sharing together as He leads us along. Bring your Bible if you have one. Your facilitator will have extra ones available in class.

Each person will set individual goals for themselves. We will share these goals and work toward reaching them together. Sharing in class is always optional.

Each week, we will have a time to focus on a health topic to keep us informed of how to do our best on the program.

We will be in a small group setting. We will all be responsible to encourage each other and keep each other accountable.

***Is this a weight loss class?***

This is a class that God laid on my heart over a ten year period. My personal journey to better health included weight loss; however, this is not just a weight loss class. The class focuses on many areas of health and fitness for ladies and their families. If someone joins the class and follows the program, weight loss will be a result. Many different sizes of ladies have benefited from this program. Ladies have come with high blood pressure, high cholesterol, arthritis, stress-related problems and all sorts of health issues. The Circle of Health that we follow will benefit everyone.

***Will we weigh?***

We will not weigh in each week; however you are encouraged to weigh in at home. Please limit this to once per week. Instead of weighing, we will be focusing on bringing down our waist measurements and resetting metabolism for those that need to do so.

***How often will measurements be taken and will we share them*?**

We will take measurements during the first session. We will take them again after six weeks and then again after twelve weeks. This will be done one-on-one, or you can do your own. What is shared openly in this class is entirely up to each individual.

***What will we measure?***

We will measure our waist.

***Will there be any other type of measurements?***

We will measure our body fat the first week, after six weeks, and again at twelve weeks.

***Will the things we share in class be shared outside of the class?***

No! We must have confidentiality in this class in order for it to be effective. We are here to pray, support, help, encourage and love each other. In fact, without transparency the class will not be effective. In the class I share many things about my life and my family. This is what God has led me to do in order to help others. Your facilitator will probably do the same. What you choose to share will be entirely up to you. Again, sharing is totally God-led and optional. What is not optional is the level of trust we must have in each other to keep things confidential. That is the only way the class will function correctly.

# My Story

I have been battling weight for over half of my life now. Almost twenty-two years ago, I was able to lose down to what is considered to be a healthy weight for me. I am 5 ft. 3½ in. tall and am a size 6 petite. For me, that is a healthy weight. That is a weight that I have been able to maintain for over twenty-one years now. However, I have to be disciplined to stay at this size. It does not come naturally. This program is a plan that I have followed for over twenty-one years now in order to maintain the weight loss. I am thankful to be able to share it with you. This is my story concerning weight.

I am one of those ladies who gained a little weight with the first pregnancy and kept five pounds of it, a little more with the second pregnancy and kept ten pounds of it and a lot of weight with the third pregnancy and kept all of it for a grand total of sixty pounds over my pre-pregnancy weight. To put it bluntly, I was getting heavier each year and I was becoming very unhappy with myself. I was twenty-eight years old, overweight, and exhausted! And to top it all off, I was continuing to gain. My lifestyle and my metabolism had slowed way down. I felt unhealthy for the first time in my life. I had zero energy, and to be honest, I didn't know what to do about it. I was going into a size 16 dress which was not something that I wanted to do. Prior to this, I had been a person who really didn't even have to watch my weight, so being on a "diet" was foreign to me.

It didn't take me long to find out that dieting was not going to work anyway. If anything, I believe that what I refer to as dieting was making my metabolism even slower. Before having the babies, I had always been very active and enjoyed all kinds of activities, but not now. I was now in my early thirties and felt old. I was going up, up, up in dress sizes and like I said, I didn't know what to do about it.

Twenty-two years ago, I decided to try to lose weight and gain control of my health one more time. This time I tried something totally different from anything I had done before. A friend of mine had given me a simple sheet of paper with a list of foods and the caloric count for all of them. It was from a local state health extension service. On the back of the sheet it gave some simple math to do to figure what you must eat in order to lose one or two pounds a week. I began going to an accountability group with her and doing the plan on this sheet of paper. The plan that I followed is the core nutrition section of this program. Having followed this for so many years, I have also included additional eating habits that have worked for me and helped me to maintain the weight loss. It is a simple calorie counting plan using a wonderful group of foods called free calorie foods to curb the appetite. Over the years I have revised the plan for myself, doing basically what works! Within three weeks, I had lost eleven pounds. Over the next ten months, I lost a total of fifty-two pounds. It was slow but consistent. Remember, I said I had gained sixty pounds. Well, I was nineteen with my first child. Now, I was thirty-two. I realized that I had reached a healthy weight for my age and metabolism that I could maintain for the long haul.

When you lose weight like this, a lot of people want to know how you did it. It is a very personal journey and unless someone is ready to do it, it is very difficult to even explain the program to them. Even though I was going to a group, I believe that God was doing a mighty work in my life as far as discipline and change, and I give Him all the glory! When my friends would ask me, I would try to help them, sometimes even writing down exactly what I ate for them. I had such a strong desire to help other people, but for the most part, it did not seem like the timing was right. I believe that now is the time. For the past twenty-two years, I have been able for the most part to continue to keep the weight off by living on the same plan. I have five pounds that I have battled from time to time, but during these years have not had to fight more than that. I am fifty-five now, and I feel great! I have a tremendous amount of energy and am able to do so many things that I enjoy. I very seldom get tired and most of the time I can honestly say that my energy level is high. Now is a good time to say all praise, honor and glory goes to the Lord. Remember the verse... ***through Christ who gives me strength!***

One thing that has helped me over the years is that I have developed a strong interest in fitness and nutrition. I have read and studied this for these twenty-two years. There are some good plans out there if you take the time to buy them, to study them, and then follow them. However, I have already done the study part for you. It has been a desire of mine for many years to help other ladies gain control of their health. Basically, this book is me sharing what I have learned and what has worked for me over the years with you. Like I said, there are many good plans out there both secular and faith based; however, most of the ones I have studied rely on a good bit of deprivation, or else they eliminate entire food groups from your diet. I personally do not believe that this can be done for the rest of your life. My plan combines five components that lead to better health, and there are no foods or food groups that are totally eliminated. I have studied strength training and have been certified in strength training. I worked for over three years, training the public as a personal trainer, tailoring personal plans including nutrition and exercise plans for ladies. I have worked with ladies one on one to help them reset metabolism. I am also a certified group fitness instructor and lead classes in strength training and cardiovascular exercise. During these years, whether I have been at the gym or somewhere else training, I have always felt a longing to help the ladies at my church and other churches and I have always felt that eventually, God would allow me to share this with all of you. Why? Because the truth is that this is a spiritual battle. Much more on that to come!

I want you to become healthy and take control of this area of your life. I know firsthand what a difference it will make in your life. I have shared the desire to write this with a very few close friends over the years and asked them to pray, because I didn't know exactly what God had in mind for me to do with it, or what format it would take. Recently, He had spoken to me and I feel that the time is now to share this program with ladies who have a desire to serve God to the best of their ability. In your groups you will encourage each other and keep each other accountable on a long term basis. This is not a short term program that will have an end. The twelve weeks are only a jump start to better health through better nutrition, hydration, exercise, and stress reduction. This is a new way of life. This is a program to follow for the rest of your life.

If health issues stemming from excess weight, unhealthy eating, an inactive lifestyle and stress are hindering you from serving Him the way you desire to, then I ask you to pray about being a part of a Fit for His Service group. We want to be our very best for Him. After all, He gave His Best for us!

# Taking Back the Control

The first step to gaining control is to realize that you are out of control. Food can become a great friend if you are lonely, depressed, frightened or experiencing anything else that the enemy may decide to throw at you. After all, food is readily available, always there for you. You already know what the chocolate cake tastes like. It won't let you down. It is unlike other addictions in that it is not illegal, it is not considered immoral, and we must be around it and have some of it every day.

Without realizing it, I had become a great friend of food in a time in my life where I was very isolated from others. There had been some huge disappointments in my family life; I also lost several close family members in a short period of time. My Daddy and two of my aunts that I was very close to passed away from diabetes and cancer within several years of each other. I was having and raising my babies during this time and I became very isolated and lonely. Without realizing it, I had allowed my lifestyle to become very sedentary and I believe that my metabolism had slowed way down. I was working hard at home every day, staying up many nights with a precious baby who didn't sleep much and taking care of my other two children and our home. This can be an exhausting existence for a young mother while at the same time not burning many daily calories. Also, lack of sleep can be devastating to your metabolism.

There would be many nights where I would be so exhausted that when I would get my family's supper on the table, I would have to go lie on my bed, turn the lights out and just lie there in the dark feeling sick and nauseated. My husband, Mike, would have to sit with the children and eat supper with them. After about fifteen minutes, I could get up and finish the day. As all moms of little ones know, supper is not the end of daily chores. There is still clean up, bath time, bed time…then you fall into bed and try to steal a few hours of sleep before the baby wakes up! This is not to complain about my precious family, as moms, we all go through those years. I just regret not realizing how out of control my weight was getting and not doing something about it sooner. You know the saying about hindsight, looking back now, I wish I had made exercise a part of my life then, I wish I had made an effort to eat healthy, I wonder about the difference it could have made in my energy level. But, God uses everything, even our trials, and if I had never gone through that, then I wouldn't be writing this!

Control belongs to God! He can handle it far better than we can. Ask Him to come and take control of your life, of your eating habits, of your daily movement. He will do it for you. Most of the time this is a process of asking Him to reveal to you the changes he wants you to make concerning your lifestyle. What is it that He wants you to get out of your life? What new and healthy things does He want you to add to your life?

When I first began to lose the weight, I did not make many of these connections in my life. I just thought I had cooked some good food and that my eating had gotten out of control. It is possible that can happen with some people, but for the most part, I have found that there is always an underlying reason when people are overeating on a daily basis. Many times it is not even overeating, it is simply unhealthy eating. There is a difference as you will see in the nutritional part of the plan. As ladies, we have a problem spending time on ourselves or doing something good for ourselves. We view that as selfish. But we must realize that staying healthy does not fit into the selfish category at all. On the contrary, great motivation for wanting to be at maximum health is to be able to care for our families.

You know, sixty extra pounds didn't just jump onto my body one day. It came on, one pound at a time, over a period of time. The same thing is true with you. We must take the weight off slowly, just like it came on. That way, your metabolism can handle the weight loss and you won't gain it back. Maybe you only have ten pounds you would like to lose. This plan can work for you. Maybe you have much more than my sixty pounds. I know that the plan will work for you. It is very overwhelming to face having to completely change your way of living. I promise you that it is worth it. You are worth it! Read God's word and realize what you are worth to Him. In the first several study sessions, we concentrate on our worth in Jesus Christ. Begin to pray as you study and prepare for the class. Ask God to open up your heart and help you realize what you mean to Him. Allow Him to peel the layers of self destruction off of you along with the weight. Go ahead and claim the victory that God wants for you. ***Galatians 5:1 Stand fast therefore in the liberty by which Christ has made us free, and do not be entangled again with a yoke of bondage.*** I have known many people who have been able to lose large amounts of weight, but I am sorry to say I have known very few who have become totally free once and for all and been able to keep it off. <u>This battle may show up on the body, but it is in the mind.</u> As you see in Galatians, God does not want us to return to the chains and bondage of anything that holds us captive. He has come to set us free! If you will choose daily to make the five components of this program a part of your life, then you will be able to be free from the bondage of excess weight. Much work has to be done, both physical and spiritual. The sentence that God gave to me one day during the time I was writing this program was: ***Anything that causes us to be less than what God created us to be, is not God's will for our lives, should not be in our lives, should not be a part of our lives.*** After my youngest son had seen that I had written that sentence, he tried to get me to change it just a little because of the grammar. I told him I could not because it had to be exactly like that; the last part has to be in there. There are some things, as Christians we cannot allow to be a part of our lives at all! What is it that you need to give up in order to be the you that God created?

It is not easy: I don't want anything that I say here to give you the impression that this is easy. It is not! It is a challenging and difficult journey. There were times when I was losing the weight that I simply had to go to bed for the night in order not to eat anything else that day. Stay strong in the Lord! You can do this. Do what you need to do to stay on the plan—go to bed, take a walk, take a bath, call a friend, get out of the house—if it is the middle of the night, have a place that you can go, get on your knees or in a chair...take it to the Lord. Cry out and ask Him for help. ***(Isaiah 41:10) says "Fear not, for I am with you: be not dismayed, for I am your God. I will strengthen you, yes, I will help you, and I will uphold you with my righteous hand."*** He already knows what you are going through. He wants this victory for you even more than you want it for yourself. What a kind and loving Heavenly Father we have!

# Seeing the Finish Line

It was not very long into my journey that I began to feel a difference in my body. The good nutritious free food, the cleansing water, the movement all began working together to heal my body from the ravages of excess fat. We really don't like to use that term, but that is exactly what we are carrying around. Excess Fat!

I did get hungry. Yes, I did! After all, I was accustomed to being pretty much stuffed most of the time. I honestly don't have any idea how many calories I had been taking in per day, but I could definitely tell the difference after being on the plan for about two days.

You must continuously have your eye on the goal or the finish line. When it gets tough, ask God to help you to see the goal and work toward it. Please set a reasonable overall goal for yourself and keep in mind that this is for life. We don't need to let magazines or media dictate to us what size we should be. A waistline that is about half of our height is a good and healthy goal for everyone. As in all things, moderation is the common sense key to setting your goals. Your lifestyle and overall health should be evaluated when setting your goals.

Set your goal and work toward it in ten pound increments. As soon as you reach one goal, begin to set your sights on the next ten pound loss. This will help to break up the journey and keep you from becoming discouraged. If weighing is a stronghold for you, that is, if you tend to weigh more than once a week, if you have become accustomed to referring to a week as being *bad* or *good* according to what the scales say, especially if you weigh yourself more than once a day, then weighing is a stronghold for you. As ladies, our weight on a scale fluctuates daily and this can discourage and depress us. That is why we do not weigh in class. Also, this can devastate a group setting because if ladies do not think they will show a loss on the scales, they will tend to skip class, hoping to make up for it the next week. This never works. Instead of concentrating on a number on a scale, simply stay on the plan, be disciplined and see what happens. I can honestly tell you that I do not weigh more than three or four times per year. My clothes will let me know how I am doing.

# All or Nothing?

Please do not fall into the trap of all or nothing. This one mindset is a lie that keeps so many people from becoming healthy. The concept of an all or nothing lifestyle is totally opposite to following the Circle of Health. If you believe you must be 100% totally on a strict diet plan and exercise regime all the time, then you will fail and do nothing, until next Monday that is! People who believe it must be all or nothing are setting themselves up for failure. There will never be a time that you can spend hours on end at the gym or eat only healthy foods. That would involve never celebrating a birthday or holiday. The all or nothing mindset is always in the future, you are always going to start a plan, usually in January, or next Monday, or after the next Holiday, or after vacation…it will never happen! Did you know that there are many people who continue to pay for gym memberships for years and never go to the gym? If you ask them, they are just about to start back, but it never happens. Instead of continuing with this never-happening, always-in-the-future mindset, why not try the Circle of Health right now? How? Go get a bottle or glass of water and drink it. You have just done one of the components that add to healthier living. Tomorrow, do another one. Go for a short walk, even if it is just for five minutes. Then the next day, add more water and do a seven minute walk. Ask God to help you reset not only your metabolism but also your mind.

***(Romans 12: 2) And do not be conformed to this world, but be transformed by the renewing of your mind, that you may prove what is that good and acceptable and perfect will of God.***

I love the way the Message Bible states that verse:

***(Romans 12: 1-2 The Message) So here's what I want you to do, God helping you: Take your everyday, ordinary life—your sleeping, eating, going-to-work, and walking-around life—and place it before God as an offering. Embracing what God does for you is the best thing you can do for him. Don't become so well-adjusted to your culture that you fit into it without even thinking. Instead, fix your attention on God. You'll be changed from the inside out. Readily recognize what he wants from you, and quickly respond to it. Unlike the culture around you, always dragging you down to its level of immaturity, God brings the best out of you, develops well-formed maturity in you.***

Be done with the lie of all or nothing! Begin eating, drinking and moving for a new way of life.

# The Journey Continues

I want you to know that I am still on this plan. I have to be! There will not be a time when I can simply let up for good and go back to my old way of cooking and eating. And the great thing is, I have no desire to go back. I choose to stay free! I only want to move forward with God's blessing of healthy living. This is what He has in mind for each of you who are reading this. I am praying for you as your journey begins. If you are in a group or even if you are doing this by yourself, you are never alone. He is with you, loving you, caring for you, wanting to shower you with His blessings. ***His plans for you are good. He wants no evil to come to you; He wants to give you hope and a future. (Jeremiah 29:11.)*** I am praying that today is the day you will choose freedom and begin the journey to become Fit for His Service!

In His Love, June Shell

# A Life of Intensity

It is only by the grace of God that I am able to share this program with you. One of the most difficult things I have ever had to do was to admit that I actually had a weight problem. You see, I didn't want anyone to know that as I was growing on the outside, I was dying on the inside. I was ashamed and embarrassed by the fact that I had let my weight get out of control. Maybe people with other addictions can hide their problems for a while, but when food is the addiction, the results are there for everyone to see.

Imagine this:

- Acting like it doesn't matter that you have gained ____ pounds.
- Having three different sizes of clothes in your closet.
- Trying to make jokes and laugh about it.
- Surrounding yourself with other people who share the problem.
- Never eating in public, acting like you don't know how all the weight came on in the first place.
- Making excuses or blaming your genealogy.
- Wearing your winter coat all day at church.
- Lying in bed at night, feeling sick and stuffed, vowing to begin a new diet in the morning.
- Feeling tired most of the time, even first thing in the morning.
- Living a life that is older than your years.
- Isolating yourself more and more, becoming introverted.
- Giving in to binging episodes that leave you physically and emotionally sick.
- Always sitting on the sidelines.
- Ignoring the beginnings of health problems that you know are weight related.

These are just a few of the things that I personally experienced or that others have shared with me concerning weight gain. This list is devastating, not only to the person that has the problem, but to their family also. Please search your heart, if you are experiencing any of the things on this list.

You may want to make a list of your own. How has weight gain devastated your life?

The first step to healing is admitting or acknowledging that you have a problem. Trying to act like everything is alright will never work for you. You cannot begin the healing process until first you admit the truth. Becoming overweight can cause deep hurt to you, not just physically but emotionally, too. It can take over your whole existence and steal the life that God has planned for you.

ACT

- Admit that you are in a battle. Admit and acknowledge that you are having difficulty. The more we let go of pride and admit that we are suffering, the more we can be free to acknowledge the fact that we are in need of help. ***2 Corinthians 12:10 Therefore, I take pleasure in infirmities, in reproaches, in needs, in persecutions, in distresses, for Christ's sake, for when I am weak, then I am strong.*** Transparency is the key to so many things, including Revival! When we finally let go of ridiculous pride, which serves no purpose but to hold us hostage, then we can finally ask for help and begin to get the healing that He wants for all of us. So, to be sixty, seventy, one hundred pounds overweight and try to act like it is not affecting us is just a lie.

- Confess to the Lord that you are in need of His miraculous healing. Being overweight is a physical illness that can ruin your life. It can affect every area of your life including your family life and your walk with the Lord. I know these things are very difficult to face, but we must face them in order to move forward. You know, at this point it is serving no purpose to go over and over how we got this way. We know how we got this way! The best thing to do is acknowledge the need, confess the need to God as well as a very few close accountability partners, and then move forward. I don't know why we have decided it is such a bad thing to confess need. It seems that we have all decided success is becoming totally self-sufficient and having no need of God, when the truth is, we are more in need of Him now than ever before. God's word confirms that we are all needy. ***Romans 3:23 For all have sinned and***

***fall short of the Glory of God.*** We need Him for eternal life and for this life also. All victories come from Him. He is fully aware of every need we have. He is waiting to comfort us and help us along the way. God's Word says that He will not only comfort us through hardships, it goes ahead and promises that we can in turn do the same for others that may go through the same things. Take comfort from Him along the way and be a comfort to others going through this same journey. ***2 Corinthians 1:3-4*** (***New Living Translation***)[3] ***All praise to God, the Father of our Lord Jesus Christ. God is our merciful Father and the source of all comfort.*** [4] ***He comforts us in all our troubles so that we can comfort others. When they are troubled, we will be able to give them the same comfort God has given us.***

- Take Action: After you have acknowledged your difficulty and confessed your neediness, then begin to take action against the desires of the flesh. We owe nothing to the flesh. ***Romans 8:12 Therefore, brethren, we are debtors, not to the flesh, to live according to the flesh.*** But we are to live in the Spirit because the Spirit of God is in us. Begin your plan of action as if facing the battle of your life. Take it one small victory at a time. When you get knocked down, cry out for help and get right back up and get going. Sometimes it will be one meal at a time, one walk at a time, one snack at a time. With God's help, you will do it!

The life of intensity is an active, productive life. It is a life spent serving God and others. It is such a blessing to get up in the morning and feel great and energized, looking forward to the day ahead. Have you found what God wants you to do? If you haven't, then you are in for a great adventure. God has special tasks for each and every one of us. As our lives go through the different seasons, many times some of our assignments from God will change, but if we stay close and listen to Him, He will always let us know what we are to do next.

After twelve weeks on this program, you will notice a difference in your desires. You will actually feel like getting up and tackling the day. You will have more energy than you could have ever imagined. Living the life of intensity involves living life to the fullest, whatever you may be doing.

The one thing that people do not like to hear these days is that there is only one way. If anyone ever tells you that there are many ways to get to God or to have eternal life, you have just been lied to. There is only one way to receive eternal life and that is through Jesus Christ, God's Son. ***John 14:6 Jesus said "I am the way, the truth, and the life. No one comes to the Father except through me."***

There are many ways to lose weight. I have seen people do it over and over. There is ***only ONE safe way*** to reset your metabolism and keep the weight off that I know of, and that is with several small nutritional meals a day, regular exercise, water, and stress reduction.

A life of intensity is a full, active life. I am blessed by God to be able to live that life each day. A life of intensity is a life fully serving God, knowing and doing what He has called us to do. It is constantly challenging ourselves, constantly growing in Him. I think back over the past twenty-one years and wonder how different my life would have been if I had not taken that journey to health. How would sixty to seventy extra pounds have affected me by now? I think of my joints, my back, my knees, my kidneys...and on and on. I don't think even I am able to fully see what God has done for me. I might think I know, but He has blessed far more than I could ever imagine. Do you realize what He is able to do for you? Ephesians 3:20-21 (The Message) ***God can do anything, you know—far more than you could ever imagine or guess or request in your wildest dreams! He does it not by pushing us around but by working within us, his Spirit deeply and gently within us.***

He will not force Himself or anything on you. This must be a decision of choice. I pray that you will choose this *life of intensity* in Jesus Christ that I am talking about. May He give you complete victory starting today!

# *Fit for His Service*

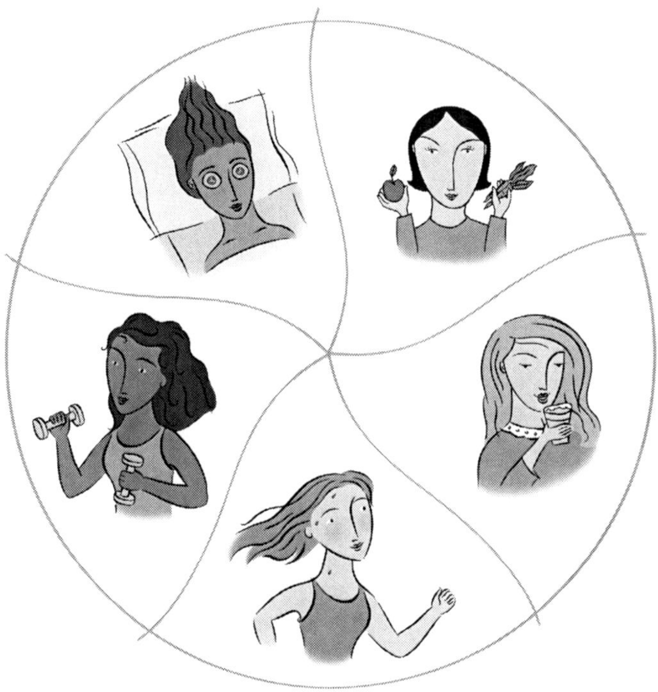

# Circle of Health

# The Circle of Health

The circle was used to demonstrate the five key components for this program. First of all, the program is very well rounded and the circle demonstrates that. There is no component on the circle that you would not want to do every week and some of them every day.

I wanted to use a circle because it stands for so many things… completion…continuation, etc. You must practice all components to get maximum benefits from the program. The Circle of Health is a visual aid that we will refer to often, so I want each of you to become familiar with it and memorize the five key components.

This is why there are no failures or disappointments when you are on this program. Each day, you will incorporate as many and as much of the five key components into your lifestyle as is possible for you that day. If you even do one component, you are becoming healthier! None of the components can be left out completely. To complete the circle, you will need to make each component a part of your life. Do not become discouraged if you have days when you are off of one or another of the components. Just remember to continue the ones you can and then as soon as you can, do the complete circle.

Here is an example so you will understand what I am saying. Over the years I have had some minor injuries or other things that prevented me from exercising for small periods of time. However, during that time, I made sure to continue with the other components. There have been times when I could not do cardiovascular exercise, but could continue strength training. When anything interferes with one of the components, ask God to help you be even more disciplined concerning the ones that you can do, such as nutrition and water, then as soon as possible, add back the ones you have been missing. This does not give us an excuse to simply go off of the program for no reason. This is simply a way to use the program realistically in our lives. This is also another wonderful reason to build muscle by strength training. When our bodies become efficient, they will not gain weight so easily and we can remain healthy until we can add back all five components.

Each time you make a healthy food choice, you are completing the circle. Each time you drink 8 oz. of water, you are completing the circle. Each walk you take, each weight you lift, and on and on! That is how the Circle of Health works.

Most important, remember we are not alone working on this. Our God is here with us, helping us and giving us strength each step of the way. I pray that the Circle of Health will become a way of life for you and even for your family as we work together to become Fit for His Service!

# *Fit for His Service*

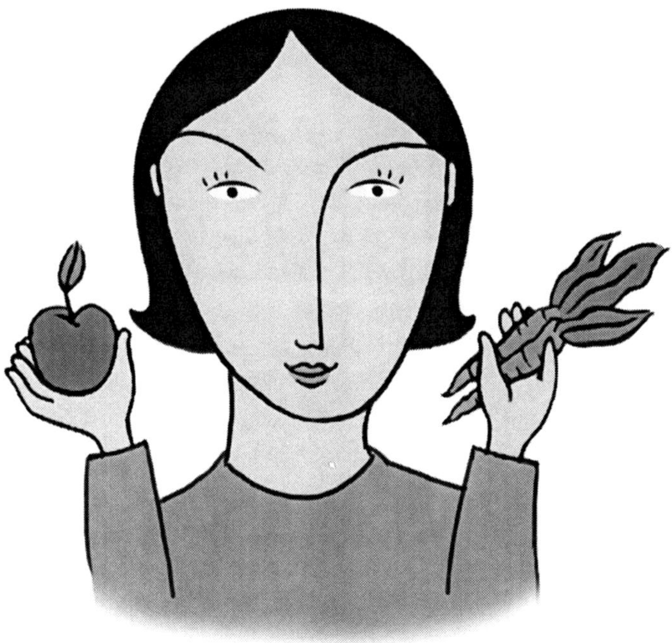

## Nutrition

# Fit for His Service Eating Program

If you have been eating a certain way for most of your life, you might think it would take a long time for your body to feel the difference if you were to change your eating habits. It has been my experience that this is not true. In fact, I have found that on a day when I am totally on the program, I can feel the difference that very day. So, if you start now, today is the day you will begin to feel a difference. It is a choice to be made each and every day. There are no specific foods or food groups that are totally off limits on this plan. This is a plan to be followed for the rest of your life. In order to do that, it has to include all food groups. That is why most diets fail. This is not about anything that you will be giving up, but the great health and energy you will be gaining. The focus has to be on long term maximum health. Of course, if you have any medical conditions that would prohibit you from any of the nutritional recommendations on this plan, you should check with your doctor before you begin and get clearance from him or her. Each individual has to figure the food intake that is nutritionally correct for them and their lifestyle. This is the plan that worked for me. Again, the goal is to eat plenty of good fresh fruits and vegetables and lean meats to become healthier. The weight loss will be a result of this. The daily recommended plan is as follows:

**1. Water**: Each morning, to set the tone of healthy living for the whole day, I recommend immediately drinking 8 oz. of water upon awakening. This begins to flush and hydrate and after eight hours of rest; it also gives me the correct mindset for the day. It sets me on a path to healthy eating and drinking. Drinking water first thing in the morning is a great way to set the foundation for a disciplined day.

**2. Breakfast:** When you begin the program, even if you have never been a breakfast eater, you will be hungry in the morning. This is good. You should be hungry. It's time to get that metabolism revved up and going strong. How do you do that? Eat and drink! I recommend that you eat your first small meal anywhere from thirty minutes to one hour after you get up. If you exercise in the morning, be sure to do it before you eat. Be sure to have water before you work out, since you have not had any during the night.

This will not be the type of eating most people are used to. You will not be stuffed after every meal. For a while, you may still feel a little hungry. I'm being totally honest. That is where the thought discipline comes into play. You must remember that even though you feel hungry, you did just eat and drink something that is good for you and also that you will be eating again in about two hours. When you eat like this, the food actually helps you lose weight, by helping speed up your metabolism.

**3. Snack**: So, we're done with breakfast. Two hours later, whether you are hungry or not, you should have your first snack and your water. After several weeks your body will adapt to this. You may then be tempted to skip this snack or to save it for the afternoon. I do not recommend that you do this. The eating needs to be spread out over the entire day to keep the metabolism going. So eat! And eat slowly. If it is nuts, eat one at a time, if it is fruit, section it or cut it into bites...give snack time the respect it deserves. Remember, you will eat again soon!

**4. Lunch**: Lunch is important. It can make you feel exhausted and tired in the afternoon or it can energize you by providing just the right amount of fuel for the afternoon. I prefer to have energy and get things done in the afternoon. I can tell you I have had times when I needed to lay my head down and go to sleep after lunch. What do you think caused that? Too much lunch! Lunch is a great time to drink a good amount of water, so start lunch by having at least 8 oz. before and then 8 more with your meal. Some people get busy and skip lunch. Don't do it. Again, stay on the plan for maximum results!

**5. Snack:** Two hours after lunch, it's time for the afternoon snack and water. You will probably be ready for this. I am always very glad to have this to keep me going until dinner. The water also seems to help curb my appetite. This is usually the time of day when I feel hungry. At this point, we just have to look back over the day and realize that we have eaten and have provided adequate fuel for our bodies all day, and remember—dinner is coming. Even if I have already worked out or done my daily exercise, sometimes it helps me to walk or move around a little at this time of day. If I am at work, I do some stretches or walk around outside the buildings. Each individual can adapt this to your own environment.

**6. Dinner**: First of all, I recommend that you drink a large glass of water before dinner and another one with dinner. You have come this far. You have stayed on the plan all day. Dinner time is here and this may be your greatest time of temptation. I can only tell you how my mind works. We cannot use dinner as a reward, or to overcompensate for the calories we have saved all day. We also cannot use it as a social time that involves going off of the plan. Dinner is probably the most important time of day to stay on the plan. This is especially true for ladies, and especially concerning carbohydrates. These will cause us to gain weight around the middle fast. It will also sabotage our goal for resetting our metabolism. So, eat dinner, but be smart. And remember...you will eat again tonight!

**7. Night Snack:** You are on a plan that lets you eat after dinner. What could be better than that? Now, about this snack… If you are hungry at night after dinner to the point that you feel you need this snack, then have it and feel good about it. However, on nights when you don't need it, then don't have it. I can tell you that some nights I have it and some I do not. However, if you are going to have the night snack, you need to have it at least two hours before you go to bed. Also, have your last water then. Nothing to eat or drink after that!

Choose an hour to cut off all eating that will work for you and your family. Be disciplined and do not eat anything after the chosen time. Make sure this is at least two hours before your bedtime. I sleep better and feel better if I do not allow myself to eat at night. Also, it sets the tone for the next day. If you are accustomed to eating or snacking at night, this will take some time to get used to. Old habits can be difficult to break. Becoming disciplined at night has to be one of our biggest struggles. This is usually when the family gathers and many times it is the largest meal of the day. However, becoming disciplined at night has more rewards than any other time of the day. You will feel better, rest better and sleep so much better when you are not stuffed before bedtime. So, when temptations come, ask God to help you complete the day of discipline.

I hesitate to write this, but I know that it is necessary for long term commitment. However, this is not permission to do anything but your very best! You will not be able to eat like this every day. OK, I've said it. There are going to be times, meals, holidays, etc. when you will go off of the plan. It is very fitting that I am actually writing this paragraph on Thanksgiving morning. Do you think I'm not going to have dressing and desert? I am! However, I am going to work out this morning and drink my water today. So, try to do the 90%/10% plan. In other words, follow this plan for what you would consider to be 90% of the time. The other 10%, give yourself permission to be off, but go right back on. Do not consider anything a failure or a reason to stop the plan. There is no blowing it on this plan. If you are even doing one of the components, you are adding to your health. Remember, this is for life! I also recommended that if you are off of one of the components that you continue with the other ones. For example, if you have a holiday meal that includes going off of the eating plan, you can still exercise and drink your water. This is very helpful both physically and mentally.

***The Food Journal:*** The food journal is important to keep track of what, when and how much you are eating and drinking. I do not want any of the journals to become a source of stress. We don't need any more things to do that take up a lot of our time. But, at least for the first twelve weeks, I recommend the journal to keep you on track. It is for your personal use, so quickly write down when you eat and what you eat, remember to include amounts, and also mark off your water intake. Hopefully, this way of eating will become a way of life and you will eventually stop the journal. If at any time you are struggling or have gone off of the plan, then make yourself journal again. It will be very helpful. Some people actually like to write what they are going to eat for the day ahead of time. That can be helpful too, as long as you keep track of it and add or take away from it as needed.

I am so excited for you right now, because I know that God wants you to be healthy and feel good. Just because you are willing to read this and are interested in changing habits, that is already a victory for you. With our God, all things are possible. He will help you through the day, and I pray that He will bless you as you begin this new way of eating. He has provided good and nutritious food as fuel for our bodies. Jesus is the key to every success in our lives. I want to praise Him ahead of time for what I know He wants to do in your life concerning your health. Fit for His Service is designed to enable us to better serve Him for as long as we are on this earth. It's not about appearance. Our ladies are absolutely beautiful in God's eyes right now! I have a vision for the ladies at our church and all ladies to be full of energy, glowing, shining His light, helping and encouraging each other, raising healthy families, all for the uplifting of Jesus Christ!

# Fit for His Service Recommended Foods and Meals

As far as I am concerned there are two types of food.

**Food for Life**: These are the good foods that God has provided for fuel for our bodies. These are foods that make us healthy and allow us to build muscle and fight excess fat. These are foods that contain important vitamins and nutrients that our bodies need. These foods not only sustain us but actually give our bodies what they need to be at maximum health.

**Food for Death**: These are foods that contribute to our aging, lack of energy, and all types of diseases. Many of them have little or no nutritional value. These are foods that have been altered far from their original state. These are processed foods, refined foods, enriched foods (that sounds healthy doesn't it?) and all kinds of packaged foods. These lead to early death or less than maximum living.

## Recommended Foods

**Vegetables:** Asparagus, artichokes, broccoli, brussels sprouts, bell peppers, carrots, celery, cucumbers, cauliflower, cabbage, green beans, green peppers, mushrooms, lettuce*, leafy greens such as spinach, turnip greens, collards, zucchini, okra, onions.
* try to choose lettuces such as romaine that has the most nutrients.

**Meats/Proteins:** Eggs (limited), egg whites, low fat cottage cheese, chicken breast, crab meat, turkey breast, ground chicken, ground turkey, turkey bacon, salmon, tuna, orange roughy. Beef* or ground beef (must be very lean, also venison is accepted). **Nuts:** almonds, almond spread, walnuts, peanuts, peanut butter (low fat or natural, be sure to read the label on peanut butter choices.)
* I strongly recommend eliminating the red meat, but if you have it, make sure it is lean and prepared correctly.

**Fats:** Fats are essential to a healthy diet. They provide much of our energy and also are slow to digest. We know we are consuming fats when we have bacon, meat, butter, margarine, and oils. The hidden fats that we also have to count are in milk, nuts, eggs, other dairy products, and ice cream. There is no way to eliminate all fats and we should not do this anyway. My recommendation concerning fats is to have most of them in the food we eat and try not to add any extras, such as butter, margarine, creams, sour cream, etc.

**Carbohydrates:** Apples, bananas, peaches, pears, figs, oranges, melon, berries, grapes, raisins, cranberries, tomatoes, peas, green peas, butter peas, beans, barley, corn, pasta (whole wheat), steamed wild rice, steamed brown rice, oatmeal*, yellow squash, acorn squash, spaghetti squash, pumpkins, sweet potatoes, yams, fat free yogurt, low fat graham crackers*, whole wheat bread.

* Tomatoes are one of the most important fruits even though they are used as a vegetable in savory dishes. They are finding out more great benefits from tomatoes all the time and tomatoes are on the free list. Fresh, frozen or canned, they are good for you!
* Use the original rolled oats. No pre-flavored packages.
* Check for the fat type and content on all packaged foods such as crackers.

## Avoid

***Avoid too much fat:*** Choose lean meats, poultry and fish. Use other sources for protein such as beans and peas. Use whole eggs in moderation. Limit all butter, creams, oils and margarine. Try to use fats that are liquid at room temperature. Spray oils are very useful.

***Avoid sugar.*** Cut way back on sugar of all kinds. Use small amounts of white sugar, brown sugar, and honey (try local). Read labels for sugar content. There are many names for sugar. Try to become familiar with all of them.

***Avoid artificial sweeteners.*** Unless you have done a lot of research and feel comfortable using artificial sweeteners, go ahead and use a small amount of sugar or honey when you have to sweeten something. With all of the artificial sweeteners as well as the oils out there, it is usually not until years later that we get bad reports on them. So, I personally don't trust anything artificial. This of course answers the question of diet soft drinks, and artificially sweetened desserts.

***Avoid too much sodium.*** This is an acquired taste. Cut back slowly until you actually prefer the taste of the food without salt. Try other ways of seasoning food, such as herbs, spices, lemon and lime juice, etc. Avoid sauces and dips with too much salt. If you use frozen dinners from time to time for the plan, watch out for the sodium content.

***Avoid eating food designed for children.*** Put away childish things. (Have you heard that somewhere before?) Like what? Well, candy, little packaged cakes, cookies and pies, sweet cereals, packaged macaroni and cheese...basically anything created for children. Mindset: If I'm going to have a dessert, it's going to be an outstanding adult dessert on a special occasion. And it would be great to even stop buying this childish stuff. Get it out of the house and out of your life! Replace it with fruit, yogurt, and other things that children enjoy. Packaged foods designed for children carry empty calories and the sugar content in them keeps us wanting more.

## Food Preparation

**Vegetables:** Choose fresh or frozen. Steam, bake, grill, sauté, or eat raw.

**Meats / Proteins:** Roast, broil, grill, bake or sauté. The sauté should be with spray oil.

**Carbohydrates:** All fruit should be eaten as close to its natural form as possible. Rice, pasta, etc. can be steamed, sautéed or boiled. Other vegetables can be steamed, baked, grilled, sautéed, or raw.

**Beverages:** Water, skim milk, soy milk (recommended for most women), tea, herbal teas, coffee.

## Portions

Portion size for this program is very important. I will use the simplest measuring system that has worked for me—that way you can use it anywhere, anytime and not have to measure. If, at first, you need to measure vegetables, fruits and grains, it can easily be done at home. Soon you will memorize what the portions look like and you will be able to do it without measuring.

* Meat...1 serving is the size of the palm of your hand.
* Vegetables...1 serving is one cup.
* Fruit...1 serving is 1 fruit such as apple/orange/pear/peach, etc.

- Other fruit such as berries, melon or other carbohydrates, etc. 1 serving is ½ cup.
- Dried fruits such as raisins or cranberries are healthy but high in sugar. Count out 10 for 1 serving.
- Whole wheat bread is usually 1 slice = 1 serving/if you eat the light 40 calorie, 2 slices = 1 serving.
- Nuts are very healthy and very useful on the program; however they are high in calories. You should count out about 10 at the time and call that a serving.
- Peanut butter or other nut spreads: use 1 Tablespoon as a serving.
- Pasta, Rice, Oatmeal, etc. 1 serving is 1 cup.

## Food Combinations

Any of the recommended foods can be used in combinations that you create. Be sure to eat them in a way that will work for you and that you will be able to continue long term. Below are a few things that are easy and have been favorites of mine.

**Breakfast**...1 serving oatmeal/cook in water in microwave/as soon as it cooks, add 1 serving frozen blueberries*/stir/add ¼ C skim milk. Coffee/ Water.
*any type of frozen or fresh berry can be used.

There can be as many variations on the oatmeal as you can think of, for example apples and cinnamon, apples and walnuts, strawberries, raisins, honey, almonds, and on and on.

Breakfast...1 slice whole wheat toast/1 slice turkey bacon/2 egg whites scrambled in Pam with salt and pepper. Coffee/ Water.

Breakfast... ½ melon, 2 slices turkey bacon/1 piece whole wheat toast. Coffee/Water.

Breakfast... ½ orange, 2 slices whole wheat toast/1 serving peanut butter or other nut butter spread.

Breakfast...½ apple/1 slice whole wheat toast/1 boiled egg/ coffee/ water.

## Breakfast Tips and Encouragement

1. Ask God to help you by giving you self control for the day concerning food intake. Mindset: you will eat again in two hours.

2. Drink your water.

3. Try different combinations. Create your own favorites.

4. Breakfast should be easy and readily available to fit your own lifestyle. Get everything ready and set out the night before. That way you won't be tempted to skip breakfast.

5. When I use turkey bacon, I cook up the whole package and store it in a large zip lock bag in the refrigerator. It can be heated quickly and tastes just the same.

**Lunch**...1 serving protein/1 serving carbohydrate/2 servings of vegetables. Water.

Lunch...small chicken breast or sliced chicken/1 serving green beans/1 serving cabbage/1 serving wild rice. Water.

Lunch...1 serving sliced turkey breast/salad made with romaine lettuce, zucchini, tomatoes (dressing is one tsp olive oil mixed with lime juice and parsley). Water.

Lunch...1 serving grilled or baked fish/romaine lettuce tomato. Make sandwich on 2 slices whole wheat bread. One serving yellow squash as a side dish. (Use 1 tsp. oil mixed with lemon or lime juice for marinade.) Water.

Lunch...1 small can tuna or other fish packed in water. Mix with one apple and dill pickle slices. Use 1 tsp. low fat mayonnaise. 1 slice whole wheat bread. Sliced carrots and celery. Use low fat dip of choice. Water or tea.

## Lunch Tips and Encouragement

1. Ask God to help you. Be prepared for lunch by packing food ahead of time.

2. Make use of a small lunch cooler.

3. Use different combinations.

4. You will eat again in two hours.

5. Drink your water.

6. Take a walk if at all possible, even for 10 minutes.

7. Be prepared for lunch by using baked chicken. I bake whole chickens or use rotisserie chickens from the store. I go ahead and cut them up and store in the refrigerator. This is great to use for lunch or even a few bites for a snack.

**Dinner...** 1 serving sliced chicken/1 small baked sweet potato/1 serving brussels sprouts, small green salad. (Dressing: 1 tsp. oil with lemon or lime juice or 1 Tbsp. low-fat dressing of choice.) Water, tea or coffee.

Dinner...1 serving grilled salmon/ steamed vegetables (cauliflower, broccoli, carrots)/ 1 serving brown rice/ small green salad with approved dressing.

Dinner...1 grilled turkey burger on whole wheat bread/ lettuce, tomato/ pickles. Side of green vegetable of choice. Water or tea.

## Dinner Tips and Encouragement

1. Ask God to help you. HE cares about all aspects of your life. You made it through the day. Stretch and feel healthy!

2. Drink water before dinner.

3. Be prepared for dinner.

4. As much as possible, let your family in on the plan and ask for their help and encouragement.

5.Keep meal preparation and clean up simple.

**Snacks...** Snacks are very important on this program. We have to have our snacks between each meal to help us stay on the plan long term.

Snacks...1 apple cut in half/spread with 1 Tbsp. Peanut butter. Water.

Snacks...½ cup low-fat cottage cheese with ½ cup of fruit of choice. Try to eat blueberries every day. Water.

Snacks...½ banana/½ low-fat graham cracker. Water.

Snacks...Mixture of 1 serving of nuts and 1 serving of raisins. Water.

Snacks...½ cup of any berry or fruit such as melon, apples, grapes, etc.

Snacks...try mixing cut up apples, raisins and nuts with dry oats. The moisture in the fruit will swell the oats and provide a filling snack. Use spices such as cinnamon and nutmeg to flavor the snack. Eat this with water.

## Snack Tips

1. There is nothing bad about snacking; in fact our bodies will work better with small frequent feedings. It's the quality and the quantity of the snack that makes the difference. This type of snacking is far from a bag of chips which has no nutritional value. Thank God for providing good food for snacks. Ask Him to continue to help you as you become healthier. He cares about us and wants us to take care of our health.

2. Mindset: Food is fuel/ snacks are actually helping you lose weight.

3. Have water with every snack.

4. Be prepared. Pack snacks from home ahead of time.

5. Try fruits and vegetables that have not been a part of your life before.

6. Keep stocked up on fresh fruit as much as possible.

## Personal Tips

1. Soups can be a great addition to salads and not be very high in calories if prepared correctly. Make a soup using your favorite choices from the vegetable list. Try to incorporate as many of the green vegetables as possible. Flavor with onions and garlic. Keep this on hand or frozen in portions to have when needed.

2. If you really feel hungry at the beginning, add more of the green leafy vegetables to your meals.

3. When you make turkey burgers, chop as many vegetables into them as possible. I like to use onions, celery, carrots, scallions, etc. It keeps things interesting, flavorful and healthy. You can make these ahead of time. Freeze them in 1 portion bags and have ready for lunch or dinner.

4. Sometimes I have to use a frozen low fat meal. Add a big leafy salad. Remember to watch the sodium on these.

5. At the beginning of most weeks, I make a soup or chili to keep in our refrigerator. The soup is made with one pound of ground turkey and

sautéed onions and all the green vegetables I can get in there. The chili is made with the same base and then I add as many tomatoes as I can get in there. I use a small amount of chili seasoning. You can season this to your taste. I eat bowls of this on and off during the week. Although the calories are very low, it helps to curb the appetite.

6. Know what we refer to as free foods and make good use of them on the program. Continue to look for and create new meals and combinations for snacks.

7. Breaking up meals is a great way to make it through the day. If you eat ½ of your lunch and do not feel hungry anymore, then simply save the rest of it for later. The calorie count is the same; however spreading it out over the day will help you to stay on the program.

8. Dressing for salads or raw vegetables: Whisk 1 tablespoon brown mustard with juice from ½ lemon or lime. Whisk in ½ cup extra virgin olive oil. Salt and pepper to taste.

**Free Calorie Foods**: Earlier in the book I said that I had used a list referred to as free calorie foods. Of course there are no foods that really contain no calories. However, the green, leafy foods such as lettuce, cabbage, greens, celery, citrus fruits, tomatoes, etc. have very few calories when prepared correctly. All of these plus more on the list are the foods that can help you to fight true physical hunger. Be sure to use them wisely and know your calorie content of each food.

This is an overview of the eating program. You may know of other healthy fruits and vegetables that you want to add in. Just be sure to be knowledgeable about the nutritional value. Also, I hope you will be creative and come up with your own recipes and food combinations. Remember, this is a life long process, and life can get long eating tuna fish and celery! I can't wait to see the recipes and meals you will create!

## Special Occasion and Eating Out

Special occasions such as birthdays, anniversaries, etc. can be tough on you if you are being too tough on yourself. The great thing about occasions like this is that they usually only involve one or two meals, even though I do try to milk my birthday for all I can! Seriously, the main thing to do is to have the mindset that the food is not the main event; the fellowship, the family, the friends, and the special times are so much more than just what's on the menu. When it's your birthday or another special occasion in your life, go ahead and plan to indulge. The next day, go right back on the plan full force..no guilt..no regrets. On the day of the special occasion, try to do a great cardiovascular workout and drink water. We try to always go walk on our special occasions. If you can, try to make walking a part of the special day.

**Eating out:** Eating out in restaurants used to be a big no when you were on any type of eating plan. In today's world, that would be almost impossible. Since we have been experiencing the "empty nest," eating out has become more a part of our lives than it used to be. Most restaurants now have healthy choices to choose from on the menu. What you really have to watch out for is the portions. They are out of control. You will almost always have to have a to-go box if you stay on the plan when eating out. It is just way too much. So choose the baked or grilled fish or chicken, with a side of steamed vegetables. Drink water or unsweetened tea and you are in control. Watch out for high calorie salad dressings, appetizers, bread baskets, cheese dips, nacho chip baskets and anything that says bar or all-you-can-eat. Share a meal, or ask for a take home box in advance. Go ahead and divide the portion and box the food to take home. Tell the waitress in advance that you will not be having dessert. If you do decide to have dessert (it better be an outstanding one!), share it with two or three people. Remember, the first bite is always the best one anyway. Mindset: After the first bite, it's just wasted calories. Also, if you have any portion of a dessert, skip your night time snack. Before you have the dessert, think and decide if it's going to be worth it or not later on tonight...

When eating out, say:

YES to. . .salads with fresh fruit, vegetables, dressings that have lemon juice or vinegar.

NO to...cole slaw, gelatin salads, cream dressings, potato salad, and macaroni salad.

YES to...vegetables that are fresh, raw, stewed, steamed, and simmered in water.

NO to vegetables that are...fried, coated, scalloped, creamed, Au Gratin or battered.

YES to meat that is...roasted, baked, broiled, simmered, boiled or grilled.

NO to meat that is...fried, stewed, braised, served with gravy or in butter or creamed sauces.

YES to soups that are...clear with bouillon, clear with vegetables, cooked in water.

NO to soups that are...cream soups, soups high in carbs, such as white potato.

**Beginning:** When you are beginning to eat healthy, I really recommend that you try to stay away from restaurants for the first 14 days. This gives you time to begin to develop new tastes and disciplines. This is also a form of body detoxification for people who eat out often. Even though you can eat out and make healthy choices, the flavors are different from the things we prepare at home. If you find yourself in a situation where you must go out and the 14 days is not up, then if the situation allows, pack your food and take it with you. If anyone says anything, just tell them you are on a new plan and ask them to be helpful by encouraging you. Tell them how important this is to you and try to help them understand that you are doing this for your health. After the 14 days, you may still find yourself needing or wanting to pack your food. You will still be able to socialize with friends and family. Soon, they will become accustomed to this and will not be bothered by it. Ask my daughter. She won't mind me telling you that for years she teased me about my eating habits such as packing my food when we went out or eating my snack every two to three hours. Then after she gave birth to two babies in less than two years, she said "Mom... put me on the program!" I am thankful to say she is now a believer and we encourage each other in so many ways.

Never let your "friends" coerce you into ordering items you want to avoid such as desserts or foods that are not on your plan. Sometimes it is more difficult for the friends and family to adapt to a healthy lifestyle that it is for the person doing it. This is especially true if you have been doing things together for years and if much of your social time has been focused on food and the surroundings. Suggest a new place to gather, like the park or some other area that is not totally devoted to food. Suggest a walk or other activity. However, remember that this is your time—the time is right for you. Your friends will need time to adjust to the "new" you.

If you are married, has your husband been your partner in crime when it comes to eating? Has one of your favorite activities been going out to eat together? Have you also enjoyed a sedentary lifestyle together sharing activities such as watching TV, computer, reading, or just relaxing?

If that is the case, again, it would be great if he felt led to go on the program with you. However, if this does not happen, let him have time to adjust to your new lifestyle. If he has never seen you spend time exercising or preparing healthy food, then he will have to have time to become accustomed to all the changes. All these changes may be difficult for him to get used to. The support of your husband and family is very important. I recommend that you have a special time, when you sit down with your husband and your family and discuss this with them. Tell them what you are about to begin and let them be a part of your journey and your success. After a very short period of time, you and your family will begin to see the results, and better yet, you will feel the results!

## The Food Journal

The food journal is important, not only for keeping track of what and how much you eat, but can also be used to track what triggers eating impulses. As we will learn in class, most of the time we are not eating from true physical hunger. There are many other reasons we eat, and when we begin to track this, we can use the journal as a tool to fight bad habits! For example: when my children were small, I never really had much time to sit down and have a meal. I was always up serving and caring for them and their needs, preparing, cleaning, etc. Then, when things settled down, I would eat my food. The problem was, I had already eaten an entire meal, standing up…a bite here and there. It all adds up. It was not until I began to write this down that I even realized I was doing it. For many people, other activities trigger eating, like watching TV or reading. It can also be other things, like frustration, stress, sleep deprivation, lack of exercise, female problems, dehydration, and many more!

So…write down everything you eat, at least for the twelve weeks!

## Holidays and Healthy Eating

Holidays are different from special occasions because Holidays are an entire season. For example, the Christmas Season really begins for us at Thanksgiving...and that's when the eating begins. Even at Easter, by the time we celebrate with two or three relatives, go to parties at our child's school, and attend all the church events, it is very easy to let go of the control. This is more difficult than the special occasions because there are choices and temptations out there almost daily. That is why CONTROL is the key to staying fit during the holidays. Here are some tips to get through the Holiday Seasons...

- Think and create a special plan for yourself ahead of time. Include time for fitness and good nutrition.
- At this time of the year, be reasonable with your goals for yourself. Try to maintain your present weight.
- Do not try to save up calories. Continue the program of eating all during the day.
- Be prepared to be offered all types of treats and special recipes that will come your way. Use control and have a bite or two of what you would really like to try.
- Let your friends, co-workers, and family know ahead of time how much it means to you to be on a plan and ask them to help you stay on it this year, by not offering things or baking for you.
- On the other hand, don't try to force your plan on anyone during this time or make them feel bad if they are not as disciplined as you are. This is a personal journey.
- When you have a party or dinner to go to, be sure to eat a healthy snack ahead of time. Do not go hungry.
- At a buffet style dinner, check everything over before you make your choices. Choose fresh fruits, vegetables and lean meat.
- If you drink soft drinks or special punch during the holidays, make yourself drink a glass of water in between every other drink you have. Make your water special by putting an unusual fruit in it. Try orange slices or lime.
- Spend more time visiting with people than eating.
- Try to incorporate your new style of food preparation into your traditional holiday meals. Serve lots of raw vegetables before each meal.
- Drink lots of water before each meal.
- Walk, walk, walk during the holidays. Cardiovascular movement is your friend all the time but especially during this time. If it's cold, even better! Bundle up, go out and walk!
- Schedule workouts on your calendar just like you schedule other things. Keep these healthy appointments.
- If you think you don't have time, then do a 10 minute power walk three times a day!
- Get enough rest during this time.
- Allow others to help with holiday preparations.

- Just say no. Allow someone else to have the blessing of bringing the cake, pie, etc.
- Be sure you are eating because you are hungry.
- De-stress: take a bath, take a break, read, meditate on scripture, take a power nap...whatever works for you and your family.
- Last but definitely not least, in fact most important of all, focus on Jesus during this time. Whether you are 6 months into this or just beginning, I know that by asking Him each day for that wonderful fruit of self-control, that He will be faithful to help you all. Remember also, there is no temptation greater than the way out He has provided!

# Meal Journal

Water #1 ❑ (check if completed)

**Breakfast** (Water # 2 ❑): Time _______

**Snack #1** (Water # 3 ❑): Time ________

**Lunch** (Water # 4 ❑): Time _______

**Snack # 2** (Water # 5 ❑): Time ______

**Dinner** (Water # 6 ❑): Time _______

**Snack # 3** (Water # 7 ❑): Time ______

# *Fit for His Service*

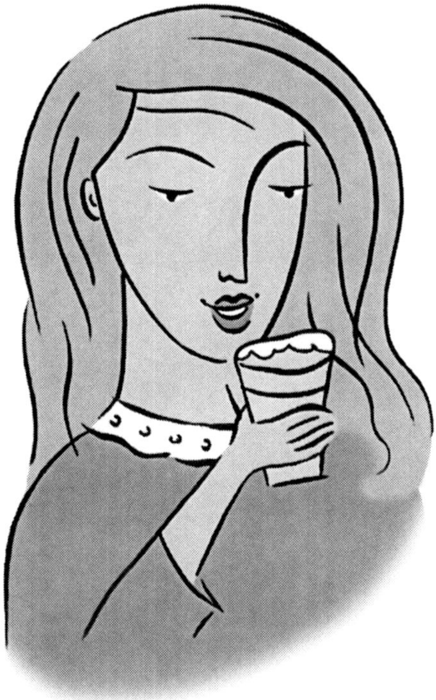

## Hydration

# Water

Water is the most important nutrient! We can live for days without food, but we have to have water in order to survive. Our bodies are made up of at least 60% water. Every organ in our body depends on water to survive. I know it is hard to believe, but most of us are walking around dehydrated. We are not drinking the proper amount of water that our body needs to function correctly. Many of our weight and health problems could be avoided if we would simply start drinking water.

Drinking the correct amount of water every day is a very important component of this program. Water is a tremendous help when you are trying to lose weight. This is because water is a very important component in resetting your metabolism. We are talking about how efficiently your body burns fat. This is a simplified explanation of how that works. The liver has many functions, but one of the liver's main functions is to convert stored fat into energy. However, the liver also has to help out the kidneys. If the kidneys are water deprived or dehydrated, the liver has to give full attention to helping them. So, the fat burning process that the liver could be doing slows down—and along with it, your metabolism and ability to burn fat. If we keep the body and the kidneys fully hydrated, then the liver can give much more attention to burning the fat from our bodies! And we like that!

Several years ago, a friend of mine came by my work one day. He had been on a healthy living program and had lost a good deal of weight. However, he had reached a stage where he was at a standstill with his progress. He began to talk with me about the situation and asked me if I had any suggestions. After we discussed his nutrition and exercise routines, which were very adequate, I asked him if he was drinking water. He said some, but not all the time. We talked about his amount of water intake and he was unaware that drinking water could make such a difference. When I shared with him the correct amount of water he should be drinking, he was shocked.

About 3 months later, he was back at our shop. It was obvious that he had been successful in dropping the remainder of his weight. I asked him what he had done. He said that the day after first coming down, he woke up the next morning and immediately began to drink his water, even taking a large bottle to work with him to use all during the day. He did nothing else different. After about three days, he began to notice a difference in his clothes and from there proceeded to lose his last 15 pounds, simply by drinking the correct amount of water. I see him at church, and he has remained the same weight for many years now. I haven't asked him, but I'm sure he is still drinking his water.

You can actually lose weight just by drinking your daily recommendation of water. That is because when we are not drinking enough water our bodies tend to hold on to it. Drinking water is an important part of our program. If you have a problem with fluid retention, this will help with that also.

At first this will probably seem like a lot of water to drink and your body will do somewhat of a flush; in other words stay close to a rest room. Soon the body will adapt to being fully hydrated. I know your body will thank you for the water. Many people that I have talked to that have reached plateaus with their weight loss or either are doing everything else right, have told me that they notice a huge difference when they begin to drink the water on a regular basis.

Water is great for the skin; it washes out impurities and will plump up the appearance of your skin when it has been dehydrated. Of course water is also good for all the major organs. Our bodies have to have water to function correctly.

Water...

* Protects our bodies' organs and tissues.
* Helps dissolve minerals and other nutrients to make them accessible to the body.
* Helps prevent constipation.
* Regulates body temperature.
* Carries nutrients and oxygen to our cells.
* Lessens the burden on the kidneys and liver by flushing out waste products.
* Lubricates joints.
* Moistens tissues such as those in the eyes, mouth and nose.

To determine the recommended amount of water, divide your current weight in half. Whatever that number is, you should drink that many ounces per day. Example: Weight is 120 lbs. You should drink 60 oz. per day. This is the formula recommended in several qualified articles online and in health and fitness books that are out today. However, this, like anything, should be done with common sense and in moderation. We have to consider several factors when deciding how much water is the correct amount for us, such as the climate we live in, the amount of daily exercise we do, and other health conditions that we may have. We are all individual and have different size bladders. Just like anything else, this can be overdone. You can actually drink too much water, so be careful to let your body adjust to this new way of life. If you do have health issues, you should speak with your doctor concerning your water intake and together with him or her to figure out the correct amount for you.

The water in tea and coffee does count as water; however the caffeine also works to dehydrate the body. You also get some water from the foods you eat.

Water is needed before you exercise. Begin drinking at least one hour prior to a workout session. Sip water all during the workout session, and drink plenty of water long after the workout session.

- Being dehydrated when you work out is not only dangerous health wise, it diminishes the performance of your workout. Thick blood cannot transport oxygen efficiently and dehydrated muscles do not use oxygen efficiently.
- Low back problems can be aggravated by being dehydrated. This is because the discs need to stay hydrated. They are more compressed when they are dehydrated.
- Muscles that are dehydrated are the main cause of injuries when working out.

So as you can see, water is very important, especially during exercise. So get a water bottle and keep it with you on this program. Soon, I hope it will become a part of your life just like the rest of the plan. You will feel better and have more energy when your body is hydrated!

On this plan, water is actually one of the key components. It is that important! The plan will not work if you are not drinking your water. Again, this is a new habit to be formed. A good habit! Let's eat right, exercise and then flush the fat out with good water.

Sometimes people say that drinking water helps to curb their appetite. What is really happening is that many times when we think we are hungry, we really are just thirsty. So drink water before, during and after every meal and snack and soon your daily intake of water will be another healthy habit that you will keep for the rest of your life.

Be sure to check off your water intake on the food journal. That is the best way to keep up with it for the first 12 weeks.

# *Fit for His Service*

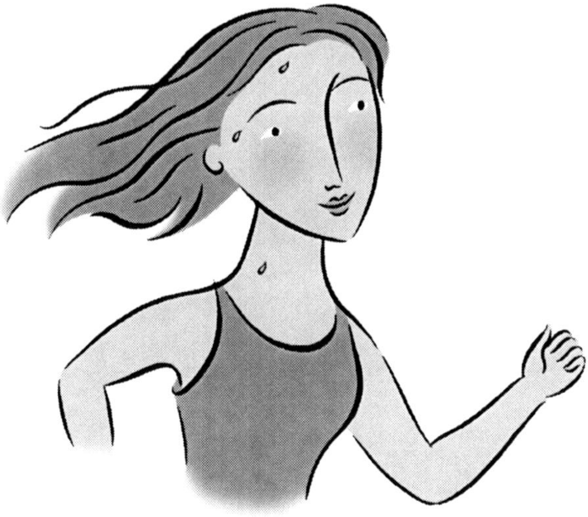

## Cardiovascular Movement

# Fit for His Service Movement

**Cardiovascular/Aerobic Exercise:** I call this section "movement," because our bodies were created to move. However, not every movement we do is aerobic. Aerobic movement is repetitive, rhythmic movement using the large muscle groups in the body. The goal for this type of movement is to get the blood pumping through our bodies. This is great for our hearts, our lungs, our muscles, and really is beneficial to our entire body. You should check with your doctor and get clearance before beginning any exercise program.

Now, we all have busy lives, some more than others. We are all doing many different things each day. I know that as a female, most days we go from morning to night, working and taking care of our families and all of our other responsibilities. However, this is not our cardio. All the things we do are great and most of them do burn a certain amount of calories, but as far as being heart healthy, those things do not count. We must get the blood pumping, reach a certain heart rate (different for each individual), and keep it going for an extended period of time.

How in the world will you find time in the week to do aerobic exercise on a regular basis? The answer is that it will have to become a priority. Remember, as ladies, wives, and mothers, we are not really geared to do anything for ourselves or spend a lot of time on ourselves. Well, I will say to you, this is not really for yourself. You are going to do this because you love those family members so much and want to be here for them. Sometimes our loving pastor asks us as a church body, "Where will you be five years from now, if you continue living as you are right now?" So, I ask you now concerning your health, "if you continue the lifestyle you have right now... where will you be health wise in five years?" Oh me! That was tough!

Let's talk about time. I believe we all have time for exercise. It is time well spent. It's a lot better than sitting in a doctor's office. Let's put it high on our list and make it become as much a part of our lives as eating and drinking. What if you can't find long periods of time every day to devote to exercise? Then use what time you do have. Ask God to help you remove the time wasters from your life. I have had many in my life over the years and one by one, He reveals them to me and He prompts me to spend my time wisely. Remember, a 10 to 15 minute walk is better than none at all. This is not an all or nothing program! In fact, as I have said before, there are no failures on this program. If on any day, you are doing even one of the components from the circle of health, then you are adding to your health and well being! Ask God to show you time for movement. I promise you, God will provide the time.

If you are really restricted by time constraints during the day such as a full-time job or other responsibilities, then early morning will be the best time for you to get in your daily exercise. Two of the classes I teach are early morning classes that start at 5:45 am. That means we get up at 4:45 to go set the room up and get ready for the participants. When I first started, I didn't realize how many people go to the gym at that time of day. I quickly found out that the early morning group is one of the most faithful groups at the gym. They come before work or before their day begins, and then they shower and get ready for work at the gym. Then they are prepared to go on with their day. At 7:00 a.m. the workout is done for the day. I love to work out early; that way nothing interferes with it during the day. So, if you have time restraints, try getting up early and doing your workout first thing in the morning. Again, this is another new habit to be formed. Soon, you will love the way it makes you feel!

Again, enlist your family to help you with this. Hopefully, some of them will even join you. You are going to be amazed at the energy and feeling of wellness that aerobic movement gives you. I am very excited for you and can't wait to see and hear the results. How long will it take for you to feel the effects of this type of movement? I will be honest. At first, you will be tired, especially at night. About two weeks into this, you will begin to see a huge difference. You will have so much more energy than you could ever have imagined! It's great to be able to move!

**What will we have if we don't move our bodies?**

- Weak heart.
- Poor circulation.
- Weak bones and ligaments.
- Flabby muscles.
- Shortness of breath.
- Increased (too much) body fat.

**What will we have if we move our bodies?**

- A strong heart!
- Good circulation!
- Strong bones and ligaments!
- Stamina!
- Good muscle tone!

# A Program of Movement

A great way to begin a cardiovascular movement program is to remember the word FIT. A good program consists of three things. F= frequency, I=intensity, and T=Time. We will study all of these in our sessions. **Frequency** refers to the number of times per week you will need to do the movement. **Intensity** refers to the intensity level you will need to reach for the maximum results. **Time** refers to the amount of time you will need to spend doing the movement.

**Frequency**...I recommend 4 to 5 times a week when you are on this program to lose weight. Three times per week is good after you reach your goal weight.

**Intensity**...You will learn to recognize your target heart rate. A good rule is that you should break a sweat and keep it. This is highly individualized and needs to be decided taking several factors into consideration. We will work this out on a one-on-one basis to be safe. Again, your doctor needs to be advised of any exercise program you are beginning.

**Time**...5 minute warm up/5 minute stretch/20 minutes aerobic movement/5 minute cool down/5 minute stretch=40 minutes total.

***Walking:*** Walking is absolutely my favorite cardio exercise. I love to walk. Now this is not your Sunday stroll. This is power walking. I have been power walking for many years and it never gets old to me. Walking is great for using the large muscle groups, great for getting the blood pumping through the veins and also a great way to get outside and enjoy the fresh air. There are so many benefits to walking. One thing I love about walking is that it is so accessible. Several years ago, my husband Mike and I went on a road trip to Colorado. We drove across country. When we stopped for the night, there were no gyms or exercise equipment available and I had been riding all day, so I would get out and walk. It was great! Walking is great for setting goals. Each year in January, I try to set a walking goal for that year. This is fun and can be done on an individual basis, with a partner, or with a group. There are several groups from our church that enjoy walking together. If you can enlist a walking partner, that is great. The time passes so quickly when you are walking with a friend. I have been blessed over the years to have a walking friend in my neighborhood. We have walked together for over 20 years. During that time, we have encouraged each other, we have done prayer-walking in our neighborhood, we have done scripture memorization while walking, and of course, we have talked and helped each other raise families. All the time, we were doing something good for our bodies!

There is a correct way to walk. You must first start out slowly, and warm up your muscles. Take long strides and make sure that every step is somewhat of an effort. Remember the game, "Mother May I"? Well, walk like you are taking the giant step, from the hip. Step onto the heel and roll onto the toe. After you have warmed up for about 5 minutes, stop and stretch out your legs (we will demonstrate this in another session). After the stretch, then begin again with the long strides walking at a pace that is good for you—at least a 15 minute mile will be your goal. Arm movement is important when walking. It is the upper body involvement that gets the heart rate up and that is what helps burn fat. So, bend your arms and pump them above the waist while you are walking. Set a pace that challenges you, but you should also be able to carry on a conversation. You will also keep this pace for 20 minutes. After 20 minutes, you will begin a 5-minute cool down, walking at a slower pace. After that, you will stretch out again, giving your muscles the signal that it is over and they can relax. Please don't be tempted to skip the warm up, stretch, or cool down. These prevent many muscle injuries. It is also important to drink water before, during and after your walk. Walking to music is also a great way to exercise and praise the Lord at the same time. Just be sure you choose music with the proper beat to walk to! There are ready-made walking program music discs out there that are great, or you can make your own with your choice of music. Either way you choose to walk, just get out there and do it! The hardest step is the one out the door. You will be so glad that you did it!

***Treadmill:*** A treadmill is a great machine for a cardio workout. If you have access to one, you are ahead of the game! Use the same walking techniques and ideas for walking on the treadmill as we used for power walking outside. A treadmill has several benefits that help you on the program. It allows you to walk in any weather (even though there are not many weather conditions that I haven't walked in); a treadmill also allows you to adjust the incline and strengthen your leg muscles as you walk. If you are walking on a treadmill, make sure it is a good one with enough suspension on it to give your steps the proper amount of bounce. Make sure it is large enough for you to take the long strides we talked about earlier. Also, when walking on the treadmill, you need to remain alert to where you are on the belt, and be careful to walk the correct pace. This may seem like unnecessary advice, but I have seen people at the gym roll off by reading or watching TV and not paying attention. Use the same warm up, stretch, walk, cool down, and stretch, when walking a treadmill.

***Elliptical or Stair Stepper:*** Either of these machines is good for cardiovascular exercise, even though I personally cannot do a stair stepper very long. However, you may be able to do either of these for 40-minutes, or at least build up to this amount of time. If you use an elliptical, try to choose one that gets the arm movement involved to get the heart rate up and burn fat! Again, use the 40-minute formula.

These are three of the cardiovascular movements that anyone can do. There are many others available at gyms or exercise groups. There are all kinds of classes that you can take. The reason I recommend these is that they are high on results and low on injuries. Also, walking is the most economical thing you can do. All it really takes is a good pair of tennis shoes.

***Group Classes:*** In the last several years, I have become very involved in teaching group fitness and believe it can be extremely beneficial to many people. Group fitness is a great way to get fit and stay that way.

Each individual must find the class setting and program that is right for them. All of your workout and movement needs can be met in group fitness classes. Group fitness provides a high level of accountability and encouragement and can turn a boring, dreaded workout into an hour of fun and movement.

Group fitness has changed from the old programs where everyone was expected to reach the same level of intensity and choices were few. Group fitness now offers all levels of activities for cardiovascular movement, strength training, balance, flexibility and much more! These classes are set to upbeat music and each participant can reach their own desired level of intensity.

# Movement Journal / Cardio

Sunday

______________________________________________

______________________________________________

Monday

______________________________________________

______________________________________________

Tuesday

______________________________________________

______________________________________________

Wednesday

______________________________________________

______________________________________________

Thursday

______________________________________________

______________________________________________

Friday

______________________________________________

______________________________________________

Saturday

______________________________________________

______________________________________________

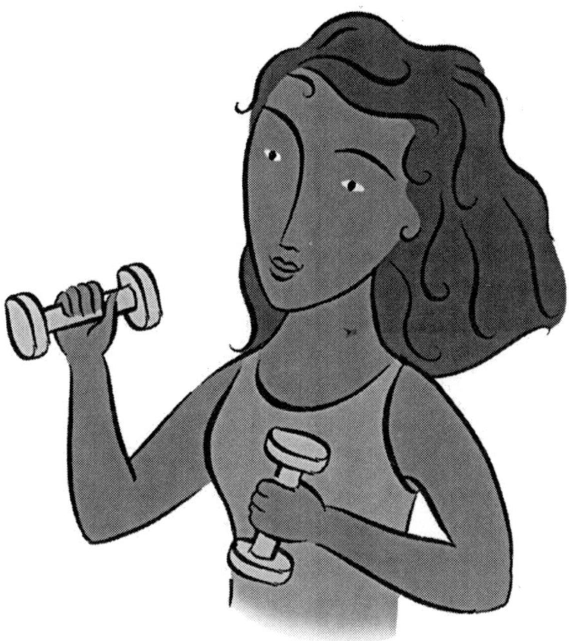

# Strength Training

# Strength Training

Strength training or weight training is something that I love to do. I am one of those strange people who are sorry when it's over because I have to skip a day in between workouts. You may say that you will never be like that, and you may not, however, the benefits to ladies that add strength training to their exercise routine are almost endless. The more muscle you have, the more fat calories your body is burning every minute, even when you are not exercising. Your body can become so efficient at burning off excess calories that you won't believe it's your body. Strength training two times a week in addition to your cardio workout is a sure way to get healthy and feel better fast. Each training session will last from 30 to 45 minutes. You should get clearance from your doctor before beginning any strength training or exercise program.

I am happy to say that more and more ladies are feeling comfortable in the gym. It hasn't always been like that. Most of the ladies I have worked with were very unsure of themselves in a gym setting, and especially in certain areas of the gym. It should not be that way. Ladies need to build their muscles and get healthy! Now gyms are actually catering to the ladies. Some have ladies' areas, and most gyms offer training to show proper techniques for strength training.

However, to begin strength training, you do not have to belong to a gym. You will need a set of barbells and dumbbells. It would help to have a bench. These are really all you need to begin a very adequate strength training program. These are my recommendations for acquiring these items.

1. Ask for this for your next special occasion. Three Mother's Days ago I asked for a punching bag. We went and picked it out from a second hand sports store and I have loved it ever since! I use it every week! Several years ago at Christmas, my son and daughter-in-law gave me a balance ball and a video to go with it. Again, I use it all the time and really enjoy it. Let your loved ones know that this is a new priority in your life and they will be happy to encourage you. People always want to know what to buy someone for special occasions. Once you become a fitness enthusiast, the possibilities are endless!

2. Second-hand sports stores are great. The equipment is barely used and the people in the store are usually willing to barter

on the price. Our treadmill came from a second hand store. It has been great.

3. Garage sales or the paper...Unfortunately, people are always selling the equipment that they had planned to use…but didn't. I am sorry they didn't stick with it, but if their weights are up for sale, you might as well help them out! (However, I KNOW that you are going to stick with it!)
4. Try a trial gym membership. Most gyms will be glad to let you try them out for a period of time. Tell them you need a few visits before you can make a long term commitment. Ask them for specials, and get the minimum membership unless you are really going to use all the amenities. Again, if you will be faithful to go, then ask for a gym membership for your Christmas/Birthday/Anniversary present.

## Basic Strength Training Recommendations

Strength training is very individualized, especially if you are a beginner. At first, all emphasis should be placed on developing the correct form or how you do the movement. I recommend that you begin training in a supervised situation if at all possible. If you are unable to do this away from home, there are some very good quality videos out there that will take you through the basics. You should not try to do this on your own because of the possibility of injury.

Rest and recovery are very important when training. For beginning ladies, you can require from 2 to 3 minutes for rest in between sets. You will also need to skip a day in between training sessions to give your muscles time to repair.

Before a training session, you should always warm up your muscles for 5 to 10 minutes walking, walking a treadmill or marching in place. Be sure to include arm movement. After warming up, stretch your legs and arms.

Training is done working from the large muscle groups to the small muscle groups.

To begin a strength training program, you will need instruction. I do not recommend that anyone try to do this on your own. There are proper techniques that must be used in order to prevent injury. I recommend that you begin with a trainer or use a good manual. I will be glad to help anyone get started. After 6 sessions, you will be able to do it on your own. We will demonstrate and talk about specific movements and techniques in class.

## Where to Begin...

Strength training begins with your large muscle groups. Then you work your way down to the small muscle groups. There is a sequence in which this needs to be done as some muscles try to assist others. When working out, follow the sequence below. I am going to explain this in terms that everyone can understand even though most of you are probably aware of the muscle groups. You will study the specifics in class with your facilitator.

## Terms Used

- **Set:** A set is a group of movements done using the same movement. The movement does not change, however, the amount of weight and the number of reps may change in a set. Most ladies begin by doing two sets of the same movement and building up to three sets of the same movement while also increasing the amount of weight.

- **Full Body:** This refers to a workout that includes muscles in the lower and upper body, including all main muscle groups. This is the workout that I recommend two times a week in order to make better use of your time.

- **Rep or Repetition:** This is the number of times you do a particular movement. Most sets include 12/10/8 repetitions. On the last two sets, your goal will be to increase the weight used. Again, form is the most important thing to remember when trying to increase weight. It is more important to keep the correct form than to do this many repetitions.

- **Range of Motion:** This refers to the extension you achieve when you are using a machine or doing free weights. You will always want to extend the muscle out completely without overextending the joint. Example: On squats, when you come back to the original position, your knees should still be slightly bent, and on any arm movement, elbows should always remain slightly bent.

- **Workout Journal:** This is a sheet you will take with you to the gym or use at home to track your strength training progress. On the journal, you have a suggested amount of repetitions to do in each set. You will keep track of the amount of weight you use and the actual number of reps you do. You will not begin by doing the amount of repetitions listed on the sheet. You will eventually work up to this.

- **Set Position:** Set position is the beginning position you will be in for any type of movement or exercise. When working out, you will always begin with this and after movement is done, you will return to set position.

- **Rest and Recovery:** The time you allow in between sets to give your muscles a rest. This should be at least 60 to 90 seconds.

- **Form and Technique:** This refers to the actual way you do the movement. This includes your posture, stance, how you are positioned on the machine, how you hold the weight in proper position, proper back support, and the proper count for the motion to take place. Correct breathing is also a part of this.

- **Count:** All action should be done with a slow count of one-two on the positive movement and one-two-three-four, on the negative movement.

- **Program:** After you become accustomed to strength training… about 6 weeks…you will begin to develop different programs for yourself to do on alternating weeks. This will prevent the body from becoming too familiar with the program and continue to give you maximum results.

# Lower Body

As ladies, our lower body is much stronger than our upper body. This is the way God created us. Large leg muscle movement is the best way to burn calories and lose weight. After you warm up, I recommend that you always begin with your lower body.

- **Leg press:** Leg press is the first lower body movement you should do after a good warm up. This is also the name of the machine in the gym. This works out your large leg muscles and your rear end.

- **Squats and lunges** have been said to be a girl's best friend in the gym, but they're also a great exercise to do at home. I have found that my body never adapts to squats and lunges. In other words, to this day they still make me very sore. That means that they are working me to maximum benefits. One of the great things about these is that you can do them anywhere, anytime, as long as you are warmed up. Ladies who have knee problems will need to modify or just do the squats. Be sure to get proper instruction first as form is very important!

- Later, when you become advanced, you can do **weighted squats and lunges**. This is where you will carry weights while doing the squat. With the squat, the weight is carried on a barbell and with the lunges, you can use hand weights. Always be careful of your back when carrying weights. As ladies, we really don't need to be concerned with adding large amounts of weight. The amount of repetitions is more important for the results we desire.

- **Hamstring Curls:** these are the back, lower leg muscles. The machine in the gym is called hamstring curl. Some of these are lying down and some are sitting up. I recommend the one sitting up if one is available. It has more support for your lower back. On this, the key is to keep your foot flexed and keep the movement slow and controlled.

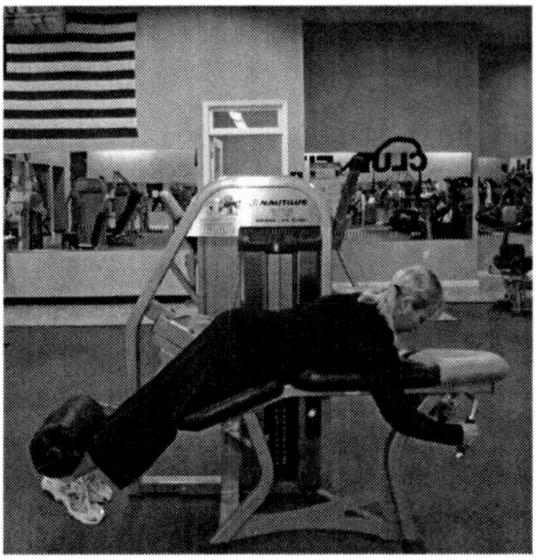

Set Position

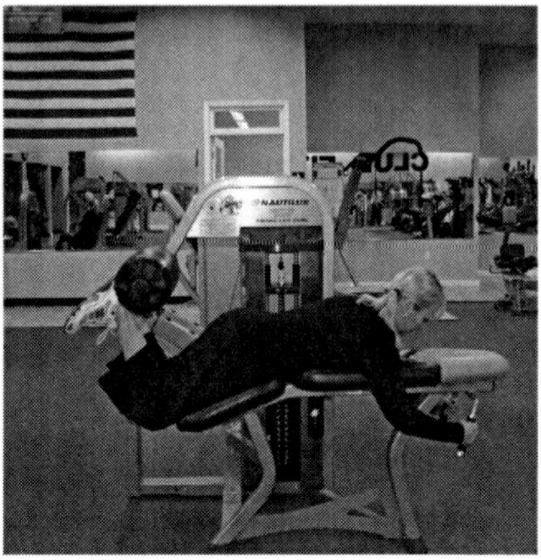

Complete Position

- **Hip Abduction:** This is a machine at the gym used to strengthen your outer upper leg and hip area. This is done sitting upright. Be sure you have good support for the lower back and use the leg and hip muscles, not your knees. Again, on this, ladies do not need to use heavy weight.

- **Hip Adduction:** This uses the inside upper leg muscles and hips. Do these on a slight recline and again, be sure to use the hip and leg, not placing pressure on the knees. The way to do this is to keep a stationary knee angle and keep feet in contact with the machine.

- **The Hip Abduction and Hip Adduction:** can be done at home, lying on your back, using your hands on the inner and outer knee to create resistance for the movement. Be sure your lower back is well supported and place hands on inner or outer knee, using resistance to open and close legs.

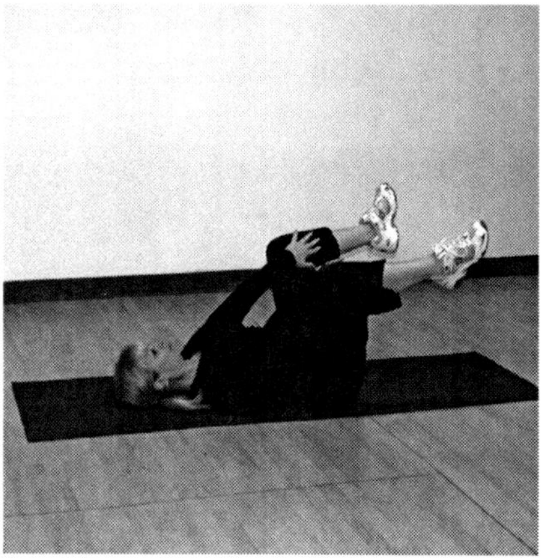

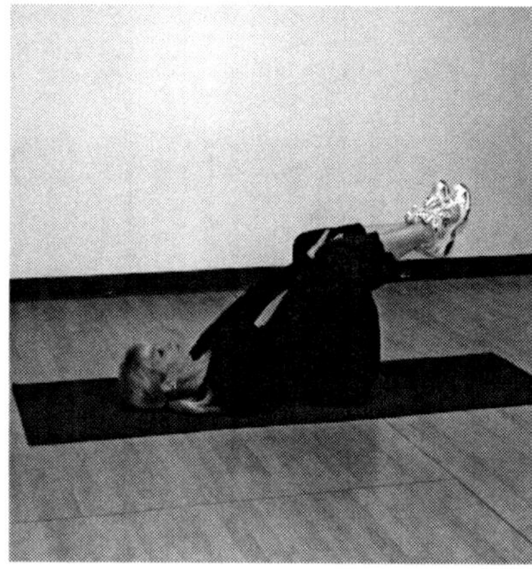

Set Position Complete Position

- **Hip Flexors:** The hip flexor is an upright machine in the gym with no moving parts. It is also used for abdominal work. This is a movement where you pull your knees up to the chest and swivel hips from side to side.

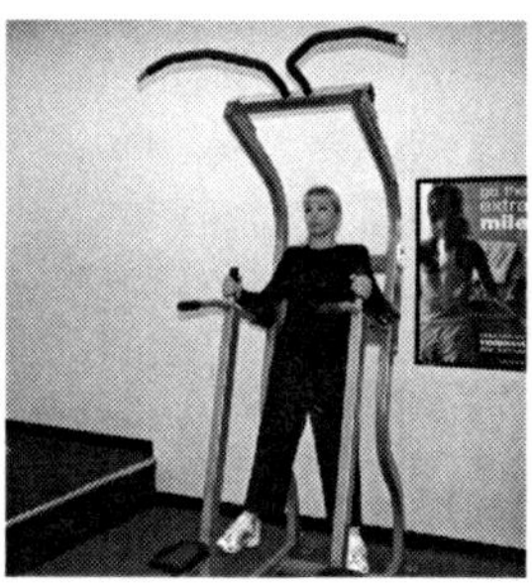

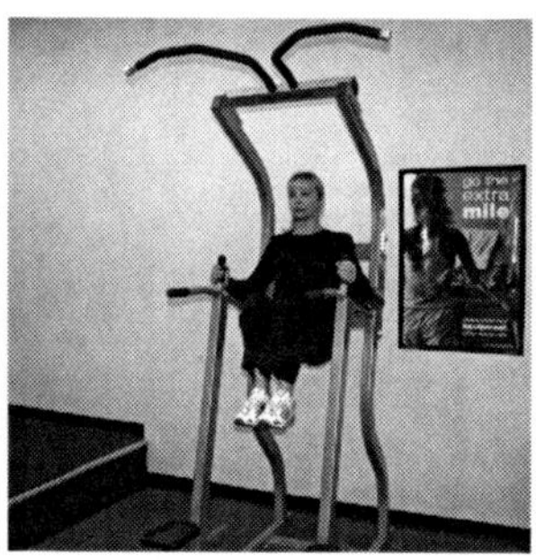

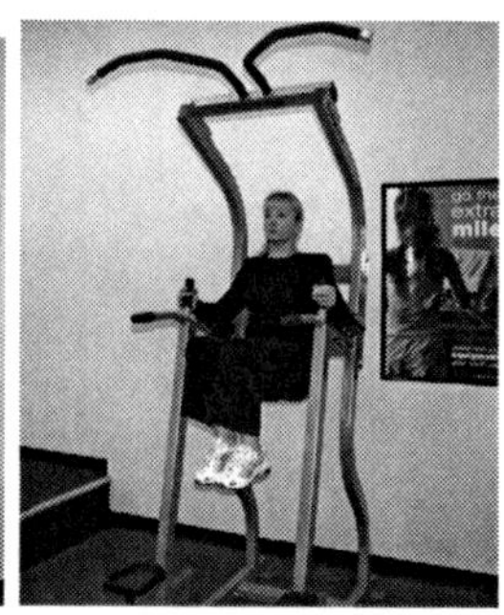

Set Position Second Position Complete Position

- **Hip Flexors:** can be done at home lying on your back. Place arms out to the side for balance. Bring both legs in a bent position and swivel hips from side to side, keeping knees together. Keep the upper body in a stable condition with back remaining flat on the floor.

- **Calf Raise:** The calf is the lower leg muscle. It will get stronger as we walk. The seated calf raise is the best machine for building a strong calf muscle. This is a machine in the gym.

You sit upright, placing the weight on top of your knees. Then raise the weight using the leg muscles, up on ball of foot.

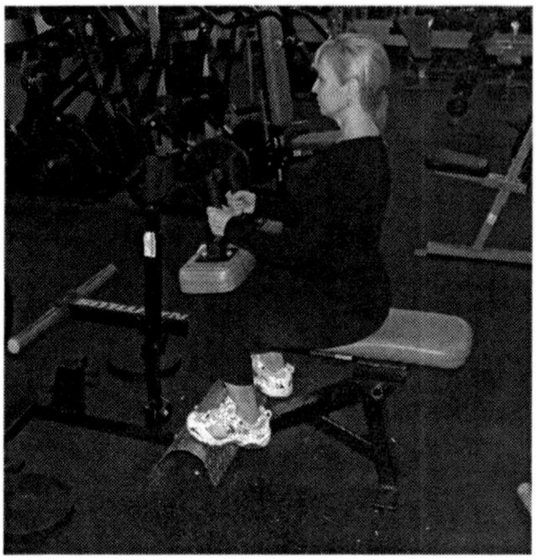

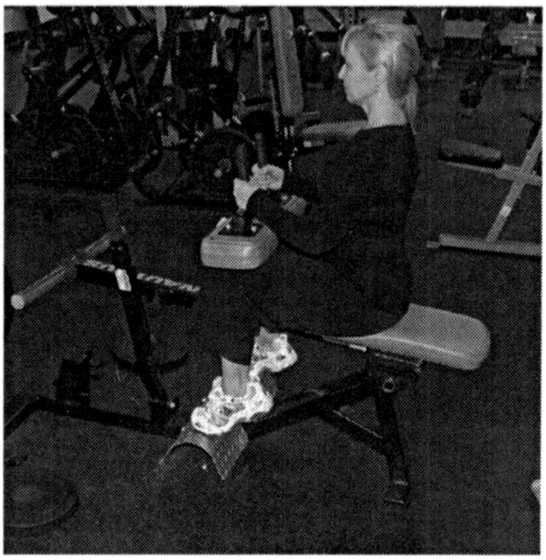

Set Position | Complete Position (Heels Lifted)

- **Calf Raise:** can be done at home sitting in a chair. Sit up in a chair with back straight. Begin with feet flat on the floor. Place free weights on top of knees, lift knees using calf muscles. Come up on ball of foot, and then slowly lower the weight until feet are flat again. You can also stand up; hold on to a chair or any support. Place one foot behind the other ankle and stand on one foot. Lift up on the ball of the foot using your calf muscle. Lower slowly and repeat movement.

# Upper Body

Upper body training is important and helps us develop our shoulders, back, chest and arms. Even though we are constantly busy, these are muscles that are not used very often. I used to say that this is why I started working out, "I looked in the mirror one day and my Grandma's arms were on my body." What a shock! Anyway, that's just a joke, but it is true that arms and upper body can become very toned with proper diet and a good upper body workout program.

- **Bench press or Chest press:** a machine in the gym used to gain upper body strength in our chest area. You lie flat on the bench with hands on bar spread out forming a V shape. Press the weight upward, on a count of one, two, trying to concentrate on your chest muscles. Then slowly bring the weight back down, counting to four, to the original position. Most ladies do this with their knees bent for lower back support. This can be done on a machine or with free weight.
- **Incline Press:** A machine or bench in the gym that is sitting at a slight incline. You do the same movement and count as the bench press, using the same muscle groups.
- **Push Up:** A push up is a good chest strengthening movement and can be used at home to replace the bench press. Lie on floor, place arms out by side, palms down. Elevate hands to increase range of motion. Use a wide hand stretch and then alternate days with a close in hand stretch to use different muscles groups in the arms, while also working the chest.
- **Pec Fly:** A machine in the gym to strengthen your chest or pectoral muscles and also works areas of the arms. Some are lying down, some are sitting upright. Be sure your lower back is supported on machine and arms are placed as if you are "hugging a tree." Keep elbows slightly lower than shoulders and press together. Slowly, let go back to original position.

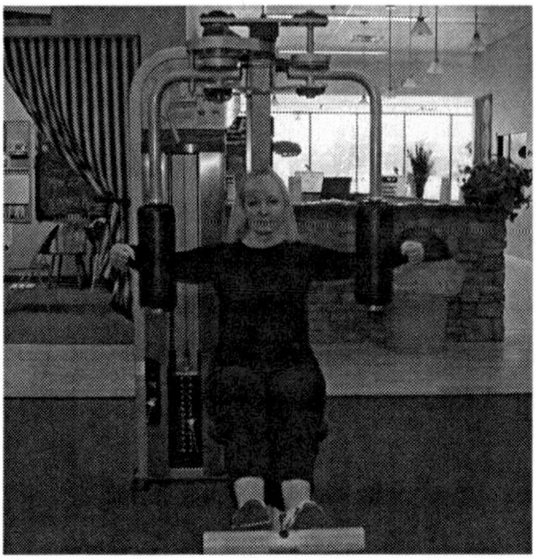
Set Position

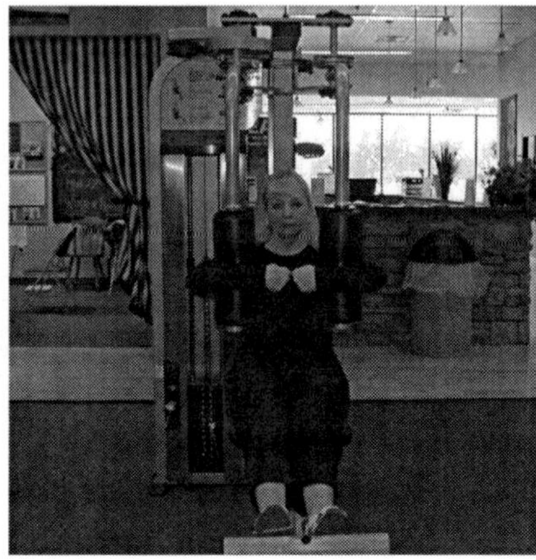
Complete Position

- **Dumbbell Pec Fly:** Can be done at home using a bench and free weights. Lie on bench and bend arms out by side holding weights with palms out and up. Hug the tree! Bring weights together and then return slowly to original position.

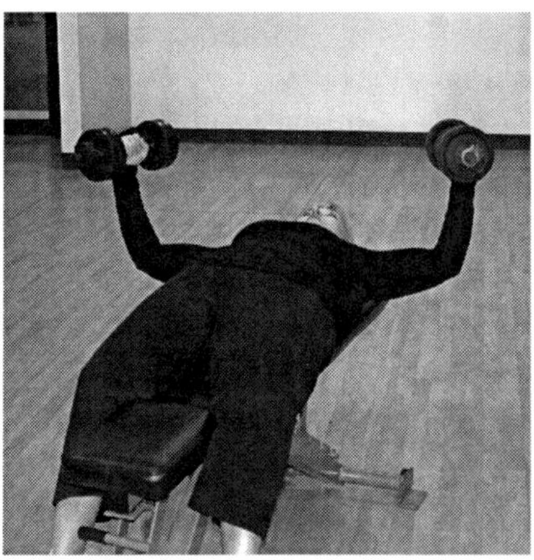
Set Position

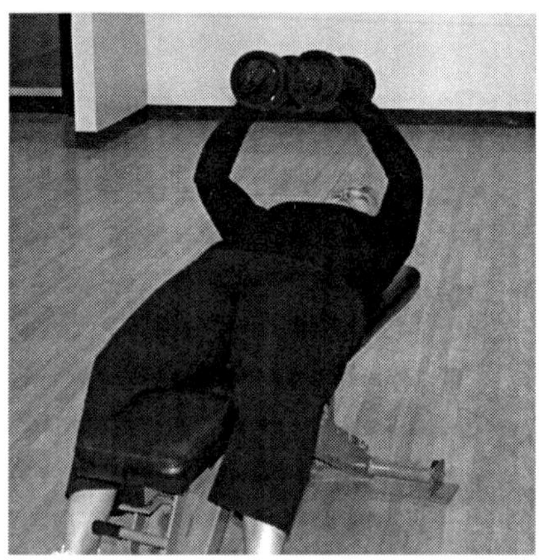
Complete Position

- **Dumbbell Bent-Over Row:** This is for strengthening the back. Use a bench and one dumbbell. Place one knee and the same side arm on the bench. Keep the other knee slightly bent and grasp weight with other hand. Keep trunk of body stationary. Keep back and shoulders parallel to the floor. Bring weight up pulling shoulder back, then release to original position.

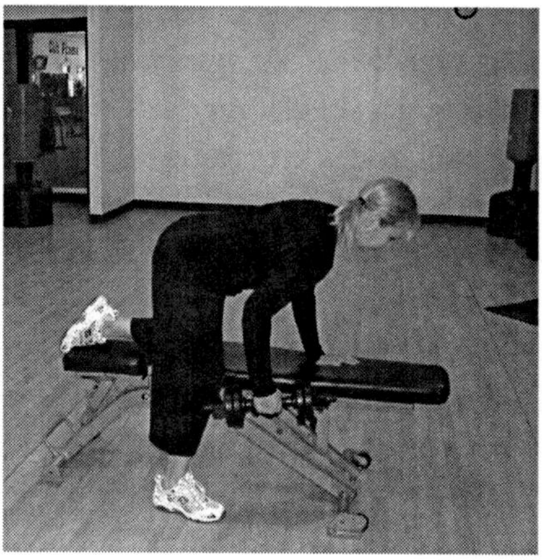

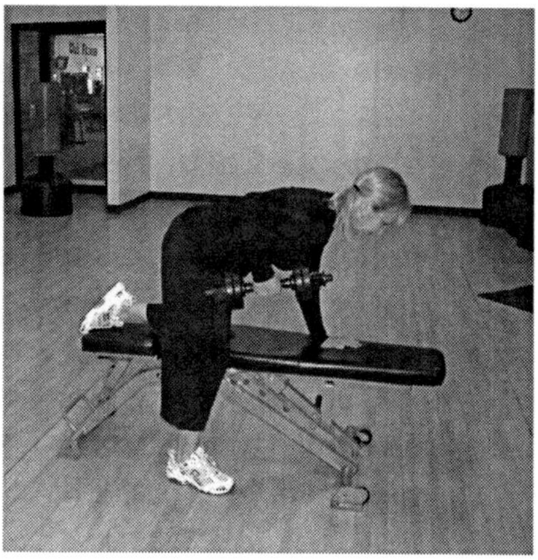

Set Position Complete Position

- **Dumbbell Overhead Press:** This is to build and strengthen shoulder muscles. Sit upright on a bench, place weights in hands with elbows bent and palms facing forward. Press overhead and touch weights together. Slowly bring back to original position.

- **Bicep Curls:** A machine in the gym used for the bicep muscles is the bicep curl. You will grip the bar and bring weight toward chest in an upward motion. Slowly return weight to original position. Be sure not to over extend the elbows and keep wrists neutral and supported.

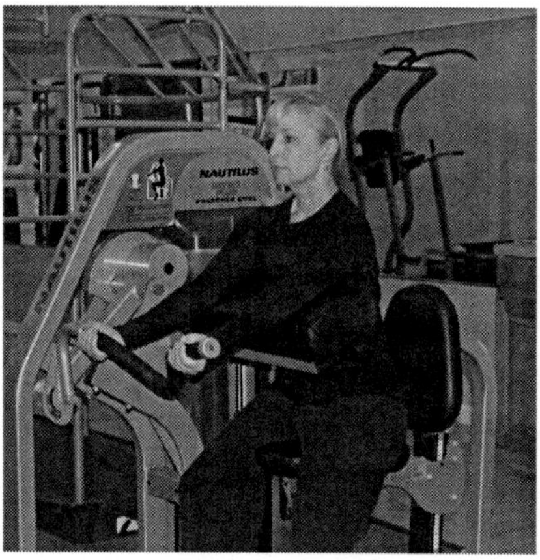

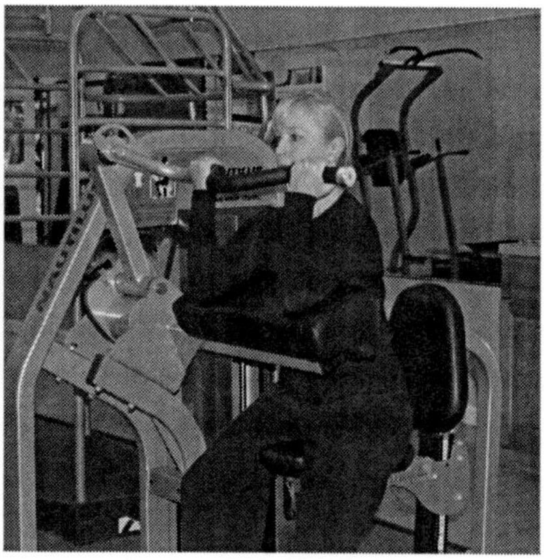

Set Position Complete Position

- **Bicep Curls:** may also be done with free weights using the same motion. You will use a bar and bring bar up towards chest. Then lower slowly back into original position
- **Hammer Curls:** For these you will use a free weight. Sit upright. Hold weight in hand with palms facing body and thumbs upward. Slowly bring weight up to shoulder, then slowly return weight to original position.
- **Triceps Kickback:** Use a weight and the bench. Keep back flat, and upper arm parallel to floor. Keep elbow stationary. Straighten arm to be flat with body, then, slowly bring back to original bent position.

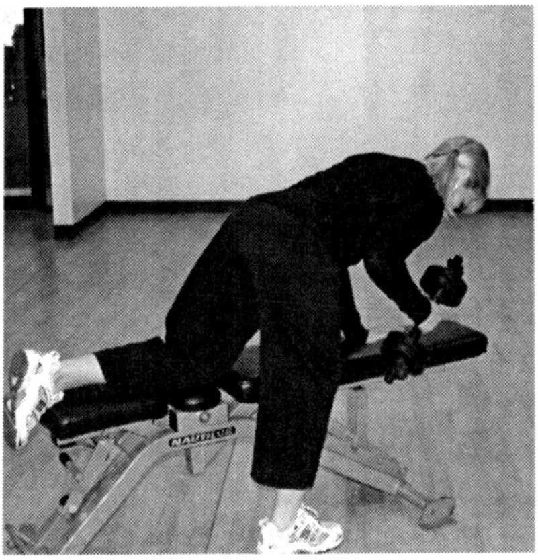

Set Position

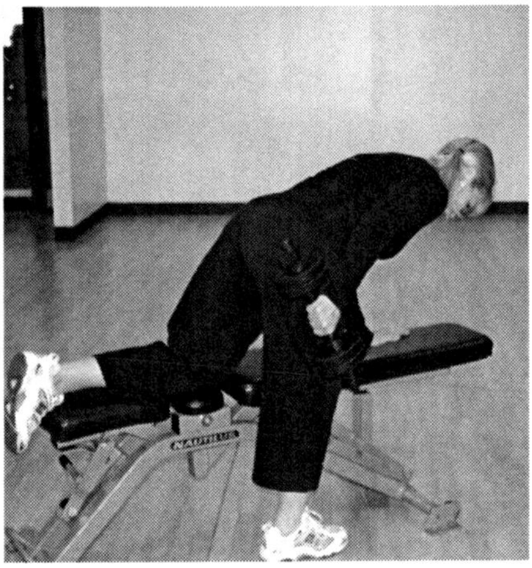

Complete Position

Needless to say, these are just a few of the strength training movements that can be done, however this is a great beginning for you to consider and the large muscle groups are used. Try to begin a program using these movements in the same order as they are listed. Begin using small weights and slowly build your strength. Begin by trying to do 2 sets of eight to ten reps on each movement. Be sure to rest for one to two minutes in between sets. Also, be sure to train two non-consecutive days per week. A good workout usually takes about 40 minutes. You will begin to feel great and have more strength than you ever imagined!

# Questions about Strength Training

I am glad that ladies have questions about strength training. I want you to ask questions. This is something that I take very seriously, because of the risk of injury involved. At the same time, the benefits far outweigh the risks and as long as our form is correct and we follow the directions, we will greatly benefit from it.

***When will we begin strength training?***

If you have never done this, and have what you would consider to be a good amount of excess weight, I recommend that you use the first month to six weeks of the program to develop a good cardiovascular program. We will work on losing at least 10% of the weight and then we will slowly begin to add weight training into the program. Like everything else in this program, this is my personal recommendation from past experience. Let's begin the cardio and nutrition program and let your body have time to drop some weight. Then we will **pump some iron!!**

***What is the most important thing to consider when strength training?***

Form! Form! Form! Technique! Technique! Technique! I cannot say it enough. You must use the correct form when training in order to avoid injury, but also to achieve the maximum results. My heart is for each one of you to learn to do this correctly. I had someone many years ago help me with this and to this day I love and appreciate what that person did for me. This reminds me of studying music. To learn it correctly the first time is SO much easier than correcting it later. So my goal for you is for you to develop your form and be a strong, confident person in and out of the gym.

***What other things are important to avoid injury when strength training?***

Hydration! You must be well hydrated at least two hours prior to doing a workout. Then sip water all during the workout and continue to drink water after the workout is done. This will hydrate the muscles and make them less likely to be injured during the work they are going to be doing. This will also help you receive maximum benefits from the workout.

Warm up and Stretch… You must remember to warm up and stretch before the workout. Then cool down and stretch after the workout.

***Is it beneficial to watch other people in the gym and learn from them?***

I purposely mentioned this because the answer is NO. Unfortunately, everyone in the gym is not using correct form and technique. Things must be done in the correct sequence, using the correct amount of weight, repetition and placing emphasis on the negative movement. This is how the muscles are built. Most people are moving randomly from machine to machine using momentum to do the work. I want you to learn correctly!

***Will I bulk up if I work out with weights?***

No. Ladies who workout with low to moderate weights and do high repetitions, will build lean muscles, which are toned. Muscles do not take up near as much space as fat and muscles are much healthier.

***Is there an age limit for strength training?***

Weight or strength training is not for children or adolescences whose bodies are still developing. It is better for them to wait a few years and then begin. If they do need to train, maybe to enhance performance in a specific sport, then they need to work out with an experienced trainer who specializes in training young people.

On the other end, adults of all ages begin to lose muscle even in their 20s. Strength training is done by people even in their 70s and beyond. One of my favorite clients was a lady who had a less than adequate bone density test. Her doctor recommended that she begin strength training. I worked with her for over two years and she greatly benefited from it. She was 73 when we began. She did gain strength as we progressed. As far as I know, she is still working out on a regular basis.

***Will I be sore or tired from strength training?***

I haven't told you an untruth yet and I can't now. Yes. You will be sore. Especially at the beginning and also when you advance to more weight. You will know that the program is working and feel great though. As you gain strength, you will begin to notice a difference in your body and you will feel so much healthier. Soreness from strength training just becomes a fact of life. It reminds you that you are doing something good for your body. Sometimes you will feel fatigued from training, usually the next day. That is why we skip a day in between, to let the muscles have time to repair.

***What can I do to help with the soreness?***

Mindset concerning this is important. Acknowledge the fact that you are doing something healthy and ignore it. Keep moving. Remember the old phrase, 'stove up?' Well, you can get that way if you do not keep active after a workout or the next day. So keep moving and you will work through the soreness. Take a hot bath. Take a power nap for recovery. Try not to get into the habit of actually taking any type of medication for the soreness. Soon, your body will adjust and you will begin to actually appreciate the soreness. It always reminds me that I am doing something good for my body. Getting sore from a workout should be slightly or moderately uncomfortable. If you are feeling something more severe than this, you should be sure your warm-up, hydration and stretching are adequate. Like I said, I want to be honest, you will never completely stop being sore from your workout. To this day, squats and lunges make me really sore. So, we'll all be walking funny together!

***Do I need special shoes or clothes to strength train?***

No. Your cross training tennis shoes will be fine. You will need to wear the correct type of sports bra with good support for all exercising. You will also need a pair of training gloves with wrist support to protect your hands and wrists.

# Stretching/Flexibility

The most important thing about flexibility training is that it greatly reduces the chance of injury. This is because stretching increases our range of motion. It is beneficial to muscles, joints and all the surrounding tissues that are so important to our bodies.

Stretching gets us ready to work out, not only physically but also mentally. It tells our body to warm up and get ready. It increases body temperature and circulation. It gives us greater range of motion when we are working out and it gets us mentally ready to move!

We should stretch every day. If we do, we will have:

- Better body motion when we do move.
- A more relaxed body.
- Reduced muscle tension.
- Improvements in our coordination.
- Strong stretched muscles.
- Fewer injuries.
- More body focus. In other words we will begin to know our bodies and their limitations better.
- Improvement and muscles preparedness for all other physical activity.
- It makes you feel good!

Just like everything else, there is a right and wrong way to stretch. First of all, never stretch a cold muscle. In other words, you must do at least 3 to 5 minutes of warming up the muscle with some type of cardio movement before you stretch it. Then, do a slow easy stretch, using slow and controlled movements. Never do any bouncing or quick movements when stretching. A good stretch should be held in position for about 20 seconds. This will seem like a long time at first, but it will be worth it. Trying to stretch farther than your body is designed to is of no benefit and can cause an injury. Each person is different when it comes to flexibility. When you see someone else bending and doing stretches, that does not mean you should try to go as far or bend as low as they do. You must learn to feel what the correct stretch is for you and your muscles. A slight muscle stretch held for 20 seconds is correct. At first you should feel slight tension in the muscle but it should go away after a few seconds. As you stretch more, you will be able to stretch further, however that is not the goal or purpose of stretching.

Breathing correctly is important when stretching. Be sure not to hold your breath when you are stretching. You should be able to do easy, controlled breathing when you are stretching. If you cannot, you should ease up on the stretch.

Remember the old saying, 'no pain, and no gain.' This is outdated and for a very good reason. Stretching should never hurt. Keep it easy, controlled, and focused on the muscle and you will greatly enjoy the benefits of flexibility.

These are a few examples of good stretches:

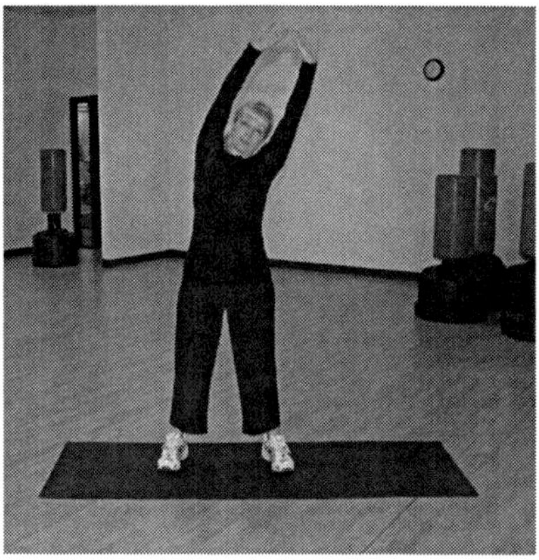

Oblique/Side Stretch

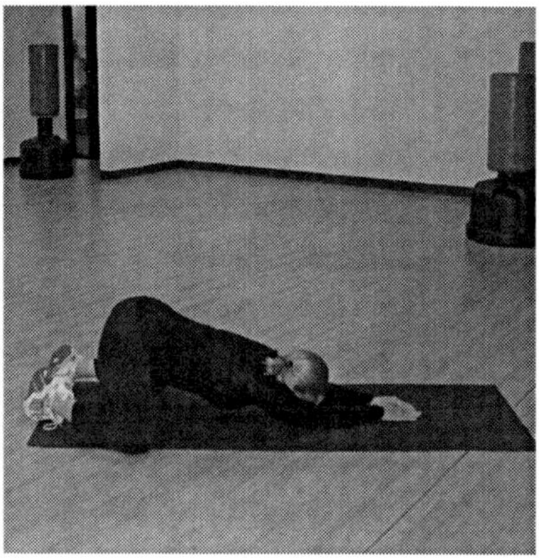

Back Stretch

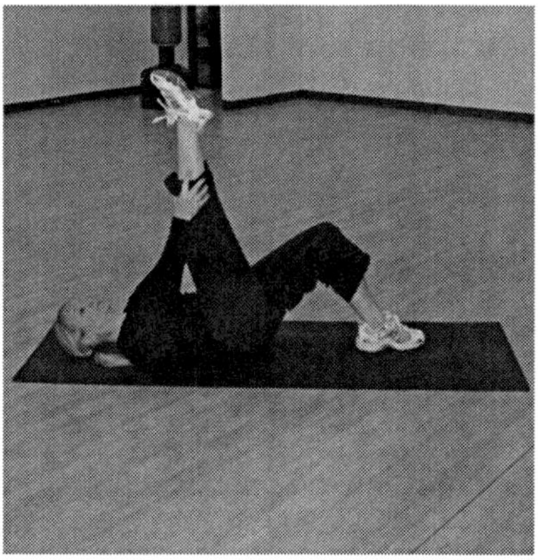

Hamstring Stretch

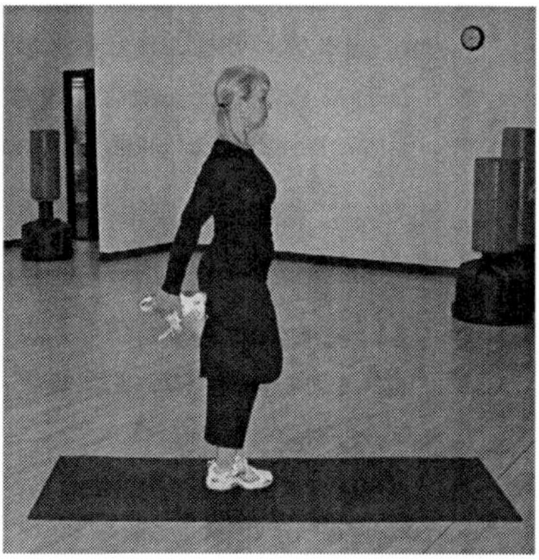

Quadriceps Stretch

## What does exercise do for you?
## What can you expect to gain from daily movement?

- Helps you control your weight.
- Helps your body use calories more efficiently.
- Burns fat.
- Strengthens your heart.
- Decreases body fat.
- Helps you lose inches.
- Increases lean muscle tissue.
- Increases metabolic rate.
- Tones and firms your muscles.
- Increases your self-confidence.
- Reduces stress.
- Helps you sleep better.
- Decreases chance of osteoporosis.
- Lowers risk of cancer.
- Increases good cholesterol.
- Decreases bad cholesterol.
- Increases endorphin levels (makes you feel good)
- Decreases appetite.
- Boosts your energy.
- Improves circulation.
- Lowers blood pressure.
- Can eliminate and help with back pain.
- Helps you encourage maximum health to your family.
- Sets a good example for others.
- Enhances your overall quality of life.

## Alternative Movement...Or other ways to exercise!

- I Hope you ***Dance***. ( I think that's a song.)
- ***Run*** around the yard with your children or grandchildren or neighbor children.
- ***Play*** on a playground with your children, grandchildren or neighbor children.
- ***Ride*** a bicycle around your neighborhood.
- Park as far as you can from the sanctuary, the grocery store, the drug store, anywhere you go. ***Walk*** as fast as you can to your destination.

- ***Carry, load*** and ***unload*** your own groceries.
- Return your grocery buggy by ***power walking*** it back to the store.
- Go on a ***hike***.
- ***Fidget*** when you are in line. Great movement for the calves. Stand on your toes and move up and down.
- Always ***climb*** the stairs.
- Alone time with your ***spouse***. (That's all I'm saying on paper.)
- ***Play*** a sport.
- Go ***swimming***.
- Do vigorous house ***cleaning***.
- Yard ***Work***... use a push mower, load a wheel barrow, rake leaves, pick up sticks.
- Try to always be aware of movement in your life. The more you move, the better you will be able to move. Remember—these do not count as your daily cardiovascular session, but they will burn calories and keep you healthy.

# Cross Training

Cross training is the best way to end the boredom factor of working out. Cross training is when you add other types of activity to your basic exercise routine. It can be anything from riding a bike, to playing a sport, to doing something different in the gym. Cross training is fun and can be challenging to your body. Sometimes we reach a plateau with our workouts and have to change them to shock the body. The body seems to be able to adapt very quickly to routines. Some ways to continue to get maximum results from working out are to shock the body by: doing your workouts at a different time of day, different days of the week, create different strength training workout routines, do fast and slow intervals when walking, add jogging intervals, go uphill or use the incline on the treadmill—anything to change it up a little so your body cannot adapt. Remember that when adding other activities, I do not recommend that you ever stop doing your basic walking and strength training. These are the two things that ladies should always continue to do weekly.

If you are going to ride a bike or do a class for one of your cardiovascular sessions, be sure that you reach your target heart rate and keep it up for the correct amount of time. Even when cross training, you should always warm up, stretch, and cool down.

Week @ a Glance. Week #.____________.
Fit for His Service.

# *Strength Training Journal*

Work out Day and Time. #1.______________. #2. ______________.

**Lower Body Workout #1.** **Upper Body Workout #1.**

## Fit for His Service Strength Training Example Workout

***Lower Body***

*Leg Press: 12 reps____ 10 reps____ 8 reps____.*

*Lunges: 12 reps____ 10 reps____ 8 reps____.*

*Hamstring Curls: 12 reps____ 10reps____8reps____.*

*Calf Raise: 12 reps____ 10reps____ 8reps____.*

***Upper Body***

*Chest Press: 12 reps____ 10reps____ 8reps____.*

*Bent Over Rows: 12 reps____ 10reps____ 8reps____.*

*Pec Fly: 12 reps____ 10 reps____ 8reps____.*

*Triceps Kickback: 12 reps____ 10reps____ 8reps____.*

*Bicep Curls: 12 reps____ 10reps____ 8reps____.*

These are sample workouts for Lower and Upper Body. A full body workout can be done as long as one day of rest is given in between workouts. Remember these are examples and there are many more movements to do. Also remember that this amount of repetitions are the overall goal to work toward. You will not be able to do this many repetitions when beginning.

*Fit for His Service*

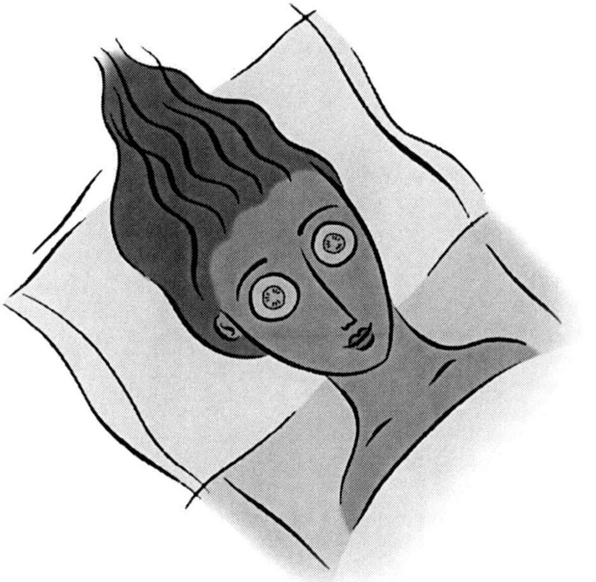

# Stress Reduction

# Stress Reduction

One important component of this program is stress reduction in our everyday lives. Just about every day I hear someone say, "I'm so stressed out," or "I'm under a lot of stress." I think the phrase under stress is a good way to express it. When life gets hectic and things get out of control, *under* is a good description of the way I feel, like I am *under* something. I feel like there is a weight of 100 pounds on my shoulders. This could come from things at work, to being too busy, to just about anything. It can even be good things. For me, most of my stress has come from needing to be three or four places at the same time. Some days, I have so much to accomplish that I don't feel that I really do any of it well. I need to slow down and regroup.

What is stress? Stress is a physical, chemical, or emotional factor that causes bodily or mental tension, and may be a factor in disease causation. There are two types of stress just like cholesterol. There is good stress which keeps us alert, up and going, motivated and active, and then there is the bad stress which is short for distress. That is when our bodies are under an attack.

So being under more stress than our bodies can handle can actually make us sick. I can honestly say that I have experienced this myself. It comes in different ways to different people. For me, when I have been under stress, I will get a bad headache or my neck and shoulders will hold tension and knot up. That is not fun.

Have you identified the causes of stress in your life? You know, we all have to have some stress, that keeps us going, but what are the areas of stress that you need to eliminate from your life? Or what things do you need to add to your life to help manage stress?

All of the components in this program will help with stress. Each one acts to help the body in its own way. For example, water helps hydrate the body. If our body is dehydrated, it is under a type of physical stress. Exercise is a huge factor in stress reduction. Proper nutrition is also a boost to the body and helps with stress. SO—just being on the program is a way to reduce stress in and of itself.

Stress reduction: Obviously, there are some things in our lives that we cannot remove from our lives. That would probably include some pretty important things in our lives such as family, friends, job, etc. For the most part this cannot be a removal process. It is a process of learning how to better cope with the important things in our lives, in a less stressful way. How can we do that? We do it just like we do everything else, **with God's help.** Looking to Jesus as our example and **asking Him** to help us.

Sessions eight through twelve will be dedicated to stress reduction. We will study and see what God's word says about the way HE wants us to live!

## Try These

1. Pray without ceasing.
2. Develop a habit of immediately casting cares upon God.
3. Meditate on God's Word.
4. Memorize Scripture. Make scripture cards and keep them with you.
5. Go to bed on time to get sufficient rest.
6. Get up on time to start the day unrushed.
7. Eat with nutrition in mind. (Stay on the plan.)
8. Drink the correct amount of water.
9. Make exercise a part of your life.
10. Get organized so that everything has its own place.
11. Simplify and de-clutter your life.
12. Develop the mindset that one is enough and sometimes one is too many.
13. Stop being a slave to things. (The more you own, the more time and energy you have to give to take proper care of things.)
14. Have extra keys to each vehicle and your house placed in hidden places. Extra car keys should be under vehicle in a magnet case. (Instead of the other purse you left at home.)
15. If you have multiples of things like books, Bibles, items of clothing, anything that needs dusting or maintaining…then consider giving it to those who do not have one.
16. Live under your budget.
17. Live in a way that enables you to pay your bills.
18. Never make a major purchase on the first trip.

19. Never make a major purchase without your spouse's approval.
20. Do not manipulate to get your way.
21. Do not take on a task, project or responsibility without talking to God, your spouse and family about it, considering the effects it will have on you and your family.
22. Delegate tasks to others when it is possible. Be sure to consider their lives also.
23. Limit phone calls.
24. Restrict cell phone use.
25. Have times with your spouse and family when the phone is off limits completely. (If it's important people will leave a message.)
26. Be a good friend.
27. Talk less, listen more.
28. Be sincere. Ask God to give you a sincere heart for others.
29. Forgive. Forgive. Forgive and then forgive again.
30. Focus on others.
31. Be kind to unkind people. (They need it.)
32. Surround yourself with Godly people.
33. Reach out to others.
34. Slow down.
35. Have alone time every day. (Even if it's just a few minutes.)
36. Listen to music.
37. Sing praise songs to God.
38. Meditate on your blessings.
39. Thank God.
40. Recall what God has done in your life.
41. Play with your children or grandchildren.
42. Play with your pet.

43. Make a list of long-term and short-term projects you would like to accomplish.
44. Work from your list and mark off items as you accomplish them.
45. Don't take yourself too seriously. Allow mistakes!!
46. Laugh everyday.
47. Cry if you need to. (Make it a good one.)
48. Spend alone time with your spouse.
49. Concentrate on the needs of your spouse and not your own.
50. ***Let God Rule the Universe! ***

# *Fit for His Service*

## Sessions

**** The shape of our bodies will never take priority over the condition of our hearts. ****

# Study Sessions

## One through Seven

Sessions one through seven deal with Encouragement, God's Strength, Commitment, Life Focus, and what God's Word says about our living habits.

1. Jesus is Our Strength.
2. God! Our Motivation.
3. Made in His Image.
4. In the Interest of Others.
5. Food as Fuel/Back to the Basics.
6. God is Love/Ask Him.
7. We Belong to God.

## Eight through Twelve

Sessions eight through twelve deal with Stress Reduction in our daily lives and how God really wants us to live.

8. Casting Our Cares.
9. Don't Worry/Be Healthy.
10. Choose the Good Part.
11. Come Unto Me.
12. Be Free.

# Session One. Jesus is our Strength

***Read Scripture: Philippians 4:8-13***

***Memory Scripture: Philippians 4:13 I can do all things through Jesus Christ who gives me strength.***

I am so thankful for Philippians 4:13. It gives such great encouragement to me! God has never asked me to do anything that I could do on my own. I am so glad that it doesn't say I can do "almost anything," or "if you try or work hard enough, YOU can do all things." That would be a disaster. On my own, apart from Him, I can do nothing! But, praise the Lord, I can do all things, through Jesus Christ who gives me His strength. With Jesus, all things are possible.

Sometimes, when a verse is so familiar and quoted so often, the verses leading up to it or after it may not be as familiar to us. Most of us know that Paul said he had learned to be content in whatever circumstances he found himself, but to be more specific, in verse 12, he says he has learned how to be both full and hungry... you have probably noticed that most of your eating habits have nothing whatsoever to do with actually being physically hungry. Don't feel bad, you are not alone. There are many reasons that we turn to food. Sometimes, we simply don't realize how many calories we are taking in each day. We are so accustomed to the way we have been eating; it has probably been a long time since we have truly felt physical hunger. Our bodies can function much better if we are not stuffed with food.

<u>In Psalms 46:1</u>, God's word tells us that: <u>God is our refuge and strength, an ever-present help in trouble</u>. If you are reading this today and you are overweight, unhealthy, stressed out, you are in trouble. If anything is causing you to live a life that is less than the one He has planned for you, then you are in trouble. Are you tied down to daily medications because of obesity or excess weight? Maybe you are underweight, but live a sedentary lifestyle. Are you under a doctor's care for health issues brought on by unhealthy living? Then you are in trouble. I love the verse that says He is ready and waiting to help. All you have to do is call upon His strength and His power to give you the ability to change your life. This is not a one time event! It is a daily process. The first thing we need to do to claim His <u>strength</u> is to acknowledge our <u>weakness</u>. We will never be free from

the bondage and hurt of anything that has a hold on our lives, until we acknowledge our need and dependence on Him. We will rely totally on Him to be able to change our bad habits into healthy living habits. It is only by His strength and grace that we are even here today. We are totally dependent on Him in every area of our lives.

With God's help, we will begin a journey together to identify the source of our hunger. We will learn to turn to Him instead of food to satisfy our needs and emptiness. During this session we will discuss what it feels like to be hungry.

Session Notes...

________________________________________

________________________________________

________________________________________

________________________________________

________________________________________

________________________________________

Write Philippians 4:13...

________________________________________

________________________________________

________________________________________

________________________________________

# *Journal Pages*

I can do all things…

Philippians 4:13

## *Psalm 46*

*1 God is our refuge and strength,*
*always ready to help in times of trouble.*
*2 So we will not fear when earthquakes come*
*and the mountains crumble into the sea.*
*3 Let the oceans roar and foam.*
*Let the mountains tremble as the waters surge!*
*4 A river brings joy to the city of our God,*
*the sacred home of the Most High.*
*5 God dwells in that city; it cannot be destroyed.*
*From the very break of day, God will protect it.*
*6 The nations are in chaos,*
*and their kingdoms crumble!*
*God's voice thunders,*
*and the earth melts!*
*7 The Lord of Heaven's Armies is here among us;*
*the God of Israel[b] is our fortress.*
*8 Come, see the glorious works of the Lord:*
*See how he brings destruction upon the world.*
*9 He causes wars to end throughout the earth.*
*He breaks the bow and snaps the spear;*
*he burns the shields with fire.*
*10 "Be still, and know that I am God!*
*I will be honored by every nation.*
*I will be honored throughout the world."*
*11 The Lord of Heaven's Armies is here among us;*
*the God of Israel is our fortress.*

# Session Two. God...Our Motivation

***Read/Review Philippians 4:8-13 (continued from week 1).***

***Memory Scripture: Philippians 1:6 Being confident of this very thing, that He who has begun a good work in you will complete it until the day of Jesus Christ.***

Leading up to this, Paul is telling the Philippians that everything he has been through so far was actually for the best because it is being used to further the Gospel of Jesus. There is so much encouragement here for us. No matter what we are going through or have been through in the past, God can use it for His purposes. I have never been through anything in my life that God has not eventually used to help someone else. On the other hand, God is always placing people in my life to help me. Even when I was struggling with weight, God placed several key people in my life to encourage me, to mentor me, to call me and keep me accountable. He even provided people in my neighborhood to walk with me. It makes a huge difference to have workout or walking partners to hold you accountable.

Another verse for encouragement is ***Philippians 1:6***. It tells us that our God will finish what He has started in us! What a relief that He will do it. Are you calling on His strength daily? The best time to do that is first thing in the morning. He will give you His power over temptations, over things that trigger bad eating habits. He will remove things that hinder you from exercising and moving in the way that He created you to.

I am certain that God wants the very best for His children, and I believe He also wants us to be our best in every area of our lives. Whatever we are doing, we are to do it in the name of Jesus Christ, giving all thanks to Him. This is from the Message. ***(Colossians 3:17) Let the peace of Christ keep you in tune with each other, in step with each other. None of this going off and doing your own thing. And cultivate thankfulness. Let the Word of Christ—the Message—have the run of the house. Give it plenty of room in your lives. Instruct and direct one another using good common sense. And sing; sing your hearts out to God! Let every detail in your lives—words, actions, whatever—be done in the name of the Master, Jesus, thanking God the Father every step of the way.*** That is what our group accountability is all about, meeting and encouraging each other as we work together to reach our goals. Have you ever been to a weight loss group where everyone sat around and shared why they could not reach their goals…so they all just told each other week after week that it was alright and continued in their old lifestyle? There are many groups out there where you are actually an outcast if you do get on the program and become healthy. We must again recognize what God wants us to be! ***(Ecclesiastes 9:10)*** ***No matter what you do, work at it with all your might. Remember, you are going to your grave. And there isn't any work or planning or knowledge or wisdom there.*** First, we must realize where our might comes from. It comes from Him, the One who wants the best for us. This is not to gain anything that the world has to offer, but He wants us to be our best in order to serve Him to the best of our ability. This involves being at maximum, long term health preparing for maximum, long term service for God. Maybe you are like so many people and have tried so many times before to get healthy, that it is getting old and discouraging. I believe our motives must be right in everything we do. We want to become healthy, because that is what God wants. We cannot do this to please anyone else, only God. Do you thrive on the attention and compliments of others? Does it spur you on when someone notices your weight loss or that you are looking healthy? Friends and family can be a great source of encouragement on our journey. However, we cannot depend on them to be our constant inner source of motivation. Eventually, the compliments stop. Soon, the praise and comments become few and far between. That is simply human nature. However, the food is still out there. The temptations are still great! It must be an inner change taking place for us to be able to continue this way of living even when no one notices. This is where the motivation and relationship with God comes to our rescue. He is with us constantly, helping us, keeping us from falling, encouraging us and wanting the best for us. He has started this good work in us.

I have a friend whose husband was always trying to get her to get healthy and lose weight. He absolutely loves her and thinks she is beautiful, but he is concerned about her health. When he finally stopped what he thought was encouragement to her, she actually did better and began to lose the weight. She was more disciplined than she had ever been. What he thought was encouragement was actually adding stress to her life. This was causing her to eat more. She also felt a pressure that somehow her husband's happiness was connected to this. She didn't want to try for fear of failure and to her that meant failing her husband. When he finally relaxed and released this battle over to her, she felt a weight lifted off of her shoulders. She was then able to give the battle over to God and became successful. It is a very personal journey for most people. Our loved ones can be a huge help, but ultimately, only God can finish this and every other work in us. It is a life long process. God will be with us along the way. During this session, we will discuss motives for wanting to gain control of our health. What motivates you?

Session Notes...

Write Philippians 1:6

# *Journal Pages*

He Who Began

Philippians 1:6

## *Psalm 27*

*Of David.*
*1 The LORD is my light and my salvation—*
*whom shall I fear?*
*The LORD is the stronghold of my life—*
*of whom shall I be afraid?*
*2 When evil men advance against me*
*to devour my flesh,*
*when my enemies and my foes attack me,*
*they will stumble and fall.*
*3 Though an army besiege me,*
*my heart will not fear;*
*though war break out against me,*
*even then will I be confident.*
*4 One thing I ask of the LORD,*
*this is what I seek:*
*that I may dwell in the house of the LORD*
*all the days of my life,*
*to gaze upon the beauty of the LORD*
*and to seek him in his temple.*
*5 For in the day of trouble*
*he will keep me safe in his dwelling;*
*he will hide me in the shelter of his tabernacle*
*and set me high upon a rock.*
*6 Then my head will be exalted*
*above the enemies who surround me;*
*at his tabernacle will I sacrifice with shouts of joy;*
*I will sing and make music to the LORD.*

*7 Hear my voice when I call, O LORD;*
*be merciful to me and answer me.*
*8 My heart says of you, "Seek his face!"*
*Your face, LORD, I will seek.*
*9 Do not hide your face from me,*
*do not turn your servant away in anger;*
*you have been my helper.*
*Do not reject me or forsake me,*
*O God my Savior.*

*[10] Though my father and mother forsake me,*
*the LORD will receive me.*
*[11] Teach me your way, O LORD;*
*lead me in a straight path*
*because of my oppressors.*
*[12] Do not turn me over to the desire of my foes,*
*for false witnesses rise up against me,*
*breathing out violence.*
*[13] I am still confident of this:*
*I will see the goodness of the LORD*
*in the land of the living.*
*14 Wait for the LORD;*
*be strong and take heart*
*and wait for the LORD.*

# Session Three. Made in His Image

***Memory Scripture: Genesis 1:26-27 Then God said, "Let us make man in our image according to our likeness; let them have dominion over the fish of the sea, over the birds of the air, and over the cattle, over all the earth and over every creeping thing that creeps on the earth." So, God created man in His own image, in the image of God he created him, male and female, He created them both.***

God loves us more than anything. He made us special. We tell that to our children all the time, but sometimes we forget that it applies to us too. He loves us!

We are made in the image of Almighty God! He had already created every imaginable creature on the land, in the water and in the sky. Then He chose to make man in His Own Image! We are made in the image of God. That is special! To be made in the likeness of the One who created us is a great distinction for us. ***(Genesis 1:26-27) So God created man in His own image, in the image of God, male and female, He created them.***

Image is huge in our world today. Every person, every organization, every business, everything you can think of has an image. Image in our world simply means what others think of us or how others see us. We are constantly striving to improve our image. There are people who actually make their living creating images for people and businesses.

So, if image is that important and we are created in the image of God, how do others see us? Do you look at others and consider them to be Godly or ungodly because of what you see? How do health issues come into the picture when we consider this?

Do you feel special? Or do you go around saying things like, "there is nothing special about me," or "I don't have any talents or abilities." This type of attitude is a great example of how we must take every thought captive. These thoughts and ideas are from the enemy to try to keep us down and out. You see, the image we have of ourselves is probably the most important! Why? Because, ultimately, that is the image others will have of us.

What will the enemy, Satan, try to tell us? This is a small list (and I do mean small, you can probably make a list of your own) of attacks he has made on those who try to change to a healthy lifestyle.

- The first lie he will tell is that you cannot do it. He will tell you that you have always been this way and you will remain this way for the rest of your life.
- When you are drawing close to God and beginning any new journey that is pleasing to God, the enemy will remind you of past failures. He will bring to your remembrance how you have tried and failed before. He will hit you in the face with the question…what do you think is going to be different this time? If this is a weight loss issue, he will remind you of all the times you have lost only to gain more back. Oh, he loves to remind us of past failures. He loves to press us down. He loves to de-press us!
- Sometimes he likes to bring up insecurities in our loved ones. It can be hard on them to accept change. Sometimes they don't even know it themselves, but they can be a source of temptation. Have you ever been on a plan only to have a loved one encourage you to just have one or two bites of something or even go so far as to tell you that you're no fun any more? They do not mean to harm you but they are feeling insecure themselves about the possible changes that will take place if you are successful.
- The tactics of the enemy are never ending, he is so desperate to keep us down that he will try anything. It is very important that we recognize and know for sure that if Jesus is in our hearts and we belong to God, then the enemy cannot penetrate our hearts. He is helpless and hopeless in that area. He can do nothing to change our eternal destination which is Heaven. With that in mind, I want you to know that the devil's main goal is to make sure we are not able to serve the Lord Jesus to the best of our ability. I believe he will use any tactic available to him to get that accomplished. That is the reason that I know that an unhealthy lifestyle is not God's will for us. It does hinder our service.

This battle belongs to God. We must constantly be in a spirit of prayer calling out to Him, asking for His help in Jesus' name. His power is greater by far than any ridiculous plan the enemy could ever come up with to hold us back.

Our image is determined by God. His word tells us exactly what he thinks of us. During this session we will discuss IMAGE. What is our image of ourselves? Is it in line with what God thinks of us? Today we will begin by reading ***Psalm 139:1-18.*** Together we will see how special we are to God.

Session Notes...

______________________________________________

______________________________________________

______________________________________________

______________________________________________

______________________________________________

______________________________________________

Write: Genesis 1:26-27.

______________________________________________

______________________________________________

# *Journal Pages*

Write Genesis 1:26-27

## *Psalm 139*

*For the director of music. Of David. A psalm.*
*[1] O LORD, you have searched me*
*and you know me.*
*[2] You know when I sit and when I rise;*
*you perceive my thoughts from afar.*
*[3] You discern my going out and my lying down;*
*you are familiar with all my ways.*
*[4] Before a word is on my tongue*
*you know it completely, O LORD.*
*[5] You hem me in—behind and before;*
*you have laid your hand upon me.*
*[6] Such knowledge is too wonderful for me,*
*too lofty for me to attain.*
*[7] Where can I go from your Spirit?*
*Where can I flee from your presence?*
*[8] If I go up to the heavens, you are there;*
*if I make my bed in the depths, [a] you are there.*
*[9] If I rise on the wings of the dawn,*
*if I settle on the far side of the sea,*
*[10] even there your hand will guide me,*
*your right hand will hold me fast.*
*[11] If I say, "Surely the darkness will hide me*
*and the light become night around me,"*
*[12] even the darkness will not be dark to you;*
*the night will shine like the day,*
*for darkness is as light to you.*
*[13] For you created my inmost being;*
*you knit me together in my mother's womb.*
*[14] I praise you because I am fearfully and wonderfully made;*
*your works are wonderful,*
*I know that full well.*
*[15] My frame was not hidden from you*
*when I was made in the secret place.*
*When I was woven together in the depths of the earth,*
*[16] your eyes saw my unformed body.*
*All the days ordained for me*

*were written in your book*
*before one of them came to be.*
17 *How precious to* [b] *me are your thoughts, O God!*
*How vast is the sum of them!*
18 *Were I to count them,*
*they would outnumber the grains of sand.*
*When I awake,*
*I am still with you.*

# Session Four. In the Interests of Others

***Memory Scripture: Philippians 2:3-4 Let nothing be done through selfish ambition or conceit, but in lowliness of mind, let each esteem others better than himself. Let each of you look out not only for his own interests, but also for the interests of others.***

God wants us to honestly love and care about each other. That is totally foreign in a world that tells us to look out for ourselves, to watch out for number one, to put ourselves first. You might say "what does that have to do with weight loss?" Well, anything that gets our mind off of our own needs and on to the needs of others will change the focus of our lives. In this group, we will not only be working toward a goal for ourselves, but helping and encouraging each other to do the same. Maybe you have already faced some difficulties in following this new way of living. Sometimes when I have exhausted myself mentally with a problem, I will share it with a close friend. I have some friends that will not just let you share and be done with it. They will help you come up with a solution. I thank God for my Godly friends. On the other hand, you can also be a help and an encourager to someone on this program…someone who is struggling.

What does God's word say about being a friend? We are to encourage each other. We are to concentrate on the needs of others. We are to care for others and treat others as we would want to be treated. None of us can go on this journey on our own without the help of loving friends.

Getting the focus off of ourselves is an important part of stress reduction. It can also be a huge deterrent to unhealthy living. This is because loneliness, obsessive thoughts of self and concentrating only on our own needs can contribute to a sedentary lifestyle. When we continue to draw inward, we are only hurting ourselves. Pulling away from others and isolating ourselves is actually a selfish act. In ***Philippians 2:7*** it says that Jesus took on the very nature of a servant. What characteristics do you think of when you think of a servant? I think of someone who is humble and busy doing all that they can for others. I think of a person who is constantly seeing the needs around them. I am so blessed to have a Mom like that. For as far back as I can remember, my sweet Mother has been attending to the needs of others. She will quickly tell you that the joy of her life is helping and serving others. She is a true example of someone who has a servant-like attitude. (By the way, my mom had her 80th birthday this year and she gets up early and power walks at least three to four times a week. She has been walking for as long as I can remember. She can still work circles around the rest of us. What a great example!)

This was proven true on my Mother's 80th birthday. I had asked all of her friends to write something about her to be placed in a scrapbook that my daughter and I were making for her. Little did we know what we would find out about our Mother and Grandmother. As we began to receive these writings from people in the mail, every one of them was an act of service that she had done for that person. They went all the way back to when she was very young. They told of visits when people were sick, of phone calls of encouragement, of gifts and giving when she had little to give. They told of many times when she provided transportation for someone to the doctor or to church. I ended up having to get two extensions of pages for the scrapbook. It is truly a testimony of a life of service to others.

In ***John 15:15*** Jesus said that he did not call his disciples servants because servants were not allowed to be in on everything. Instead, He called them friends which meant that they had full access to everything that He did. The same is true for us. All we have to do is call on the name of Jesus and we have full access to the Father, our Father.

During this session, we will discuss Godly friendship and how we can help each other to continue to stay on the program:

Session Notes...

______________________________________________

______________________________________________

______________________________________________

______________________________________________

______________________________________________

______________________________________________

Write Philippians 2:3-4

______________________________________________

______________________________________________

# *Journal Pages*

Pray for a friend

Write… Philippians 2:3-4

*Ephesians 3:14-19*

*14 For this cause I bow my knees unto the Father of our Lord Jesus Christ,*

*15 from whom the whole family in Heaven and earth is named,*

*16 that He would grant you, according to the riches of His glory, to be strengthened with might by His Spirit in the inner man;*

*17 that Christ may dwell in your hearts by faith; that ye, being rooted and grounded in love,*

*18 may be able to comprehend with all saints what is the breadth and length and depth and height,*

*19 and to know the love of Christ, which surpasseth knowledge, that ye might be filled with all the fullness of God.*

# Session Five. Food as Fuel/Back to the Basics.

***Memory Scripture: Genesis 1:29 And God said, "See, I have given you every herb that yields seed which is on the face of the earth, and every tree whose fruit yields seed; to you it shall be for food."***

God has provided wonderful food for us to eat. In ***Genesis 2:8***, God planted a garden. He meant it for man to eat. In ***Genesis 2:9***, He made it to be pleasant to the sight and good for food. As far as I know, this was the first food created. God meets all of our needs. The food He created was perfect. Daniel asked for vegetables and water in ***Daniel 1:12***. Again, it was the perfect food. After just 10 days, Daniel and his friends were visibly healthier that the other young men.

How much do you focus on food? Are you constantly thinking about dieting and food choices? How many diet programs have you bought over the years? Are you constantly searching for new plans to go on? Have you ever considered that this is a form of bondage? It is! Anything that consumes our thought life and takes the focus off of God and our service to Him is not healthy for us. If we are always thinking about what we are or what we are not going to eat, then food is still holding us hostage. It doesn't matter how much we weigh. It is still the main focus of our lives. It is still ruling our lives. We should have no unnatural attachments to anything, such as when we are consumed with counting calories or weighing all during the day. We can even take exercise too far. We are to be moderate and disciplined in all things.

I love it when food becomes simple fuel and I do not even have to think about it. God has allowed me to have the great joy of having several different passions in my life. When I am involved in one of these activities, I usually forget to eat. It is the last thing on my mind. When I am working on this program or making a plan for a client, time will pass by and before you know it, I have skipped a feeding time. I will quickly eat a bite and then go right back to what I was doing. When I sit at the piano or work with the choir or children's choir, food or my stomach is the last thing on my mind.

I hope you have found your passion. What a blessing! If you haven't been able to do this yet, ask God to reveal to you what it is HE wants your passion to be. Of course, He must be first in all of our lives, then our families, husbands first if you are married, then the children.

Passions are a blessing from God. This is where the *Life of Intensity* comes into play. Idle, sedentary time is an enemy to us. Do not become confused about this and simply busy yourself with more activity. We do not need more activities in our lives. What we all need is God-ordained passions that lead to service for Him and the uplifting of His kingdom. Ask God to help you find whatever it is that makes you literally forget to eat! Do I want you to forget to eat? No! You get the idea.

In this session, we will discuss finding out what our passions are and how that can help us to use food for fuel and nothing else:

Session Notes...

________________________________________________

________________________________________________

________________________________________________

________________________________________________

________________________________________________

________________________________________________

Write Genesis 1:29

________________________________________________

________________________________________________

# Journal Pages

Write…Genesis 1:29

## *Psalm 136*

*1 Give thanks to the LORD, for he is good.*
*His love endures forever.*
*2 Give thanks to the God of gods.*
*His love endures forever.*
*3 Give thanks to the Lord of lords:*
*His love endures forever.*
*4 to him who alone does great wonders,*
*His love endures forever.*
*5 who by his understanding made the heavens,*
*His love endures forever.*
*6 who spread out the earth upon the waters,*
*His love endures forever.*
*7 who made the great lights—*
*His love endures forever.*
*8 the sun to govern the day,*
*His love endures forever.*
*9 the moon and stars to govern the night;*
*His love endures forever.*
*10 to him who struck down the firstborn of Egypt*
*His love endures forever.*
*11 and brought Israel out from among them*
*His love endures forever.*
*12 with a mighty hand and outstretched arm;*
*His love endures forever.*
*13 to him who divided the Red Sea asunder*
*His love endures forever.*
*14 and brought Israel through the midst of it,*
*His love endures forever.*
*15 but swept Pharaoh and his army into the Red Sea;*
*His love endures forever.*
*16 to him who led his people through the desert,*
*His love endures forever.*
*17 who struck down great kings,*
*His love endures forever.*
*18 and killed mighty kings—*
*His love endures forever.*

*[19] Sihon king of the Amorites*
*His love endures forever.*
*[20] and Og king of Bashan—*
*His love endures forever.*

*[21] and gave their land as an inheritance,*
*His love endures forever.*
*[22] an inheritance to his servant Israel;*
*His love endures forever.*
*[23] to the One who remembered us in our low estate*
*His love endures forever.*
*24 and freed us from our enemies,*
*His love endures forever.*
*[25] and who gives food to every creature.*
*His love endures forever.*
*[26] Give thanks to the God of heaven.*
*His love endures forever.*

# Session Six. God is Love/Ask Him.

***Memory Scripture: 1 John 5:14-15 Now this is the confidence that we have in Him, that if we ask anything according to His will, He hears us. And if we know that He hears us, whatever we ask, we know that we have petitions that we have asked of Him.***

As we have been learning, God wants the best for each of us. He loves us and cares about us. God is providing, helping and carrying us through this program of change. Our bodies belong to God. We are to be glorifying God in our bodies and in our spirits. Our bodies are the temple of God. We represent Him in everything we do. This includes our lifestyle concerning our health. As we continue to set goals for ourselves, we are going to ask God to reveal to us what He would have those goals to be. Remember, this is not just about weight. Did you know that many of our young ladies struggle with smoking? Don't be shocked! They do not want to do it. They hate it! They have become addicted physically, and emotionally. Most of them started doing it to control their weight. There are many other things going on to control weight that are not in God's will for our lives. We must begin to recognize these and set the example for our young ladies and girls. I have had ladies in class struggling with all different types of eating disorders. There may be other things that God wants us to give up, or take up to become healthier. We need to ask God to do a revealing, first in ourselves. What is it that He wants to get out of our life that is hindering our health and our walk with Him? Or on the other side of that, what needs to be added to our lives to glorify God?

We hear and see so much these days about makeovers. Everyone wants a makeover of one kind or another. It's either a full body or from the neck up or a complete home makeover. It is fun to see the before and after. You see a run down, old house that looks like it's about to fall to the ground. Then they show a little construction and in less than an hour you see a true show place of a home complete with all the accessories. Or either it's a person who is completely remade to look twenty years younger, and again we get to see the results in less than an hour. What we don't see is what happens in the middle. I cannot imagine the pain, infection and risk that goes along with these surgeries. And the construction that goes into a huge home makeover takes months and sometimes years. We are definitely into instant gratification these days. But healthy living, by eating nutritional meals, being disciplined with our exercise, drinking water and all of these are not quick fixes.

Have you ever really had anything worthwhile in your life that wasn't a struggle of some kind or another? I haven't! I wonder what it would be like if this came easily to us. Everything worthwhile takes time and effort. God wants us to work through the process.

Have you ever seen documentaries on people who have gone through weight loss surgeries, such as bypass surgery where the stomach is restricted and they can only eat small amounts for the rest of their lives? The ones that I have seen on television or read about were really sad, because many of the people did lose large amounts of weight, but they quickly turned to other addictions. This was because they did not go through the process. They did not uncover the root reason for their original problem. Physically, they could no longer eat large amounts, so not knowing what to do with their emotions, they turned to other vices. When they had proper counseling, it worked out so much better. So, when you are on the journey, don't try to rush things. Allow God to do the work that He has started. Not only allow Him, but ask Him to reveal and heal!

The most difficult things in life such as our marriages, our families, our children, our careers are the ones we struggle with the most. That makes us appreciate them all the more. Think of the joy and sense of accomplishment when that baby is born or when you have worked out a family problem. The same is true with the journey to health. Thank God for the journey itself! Don't be in such a hurry! Take it one step, one healthy meal, one glass of water, one power walk at a time.

Allow God to go deep inside and show you why you are unhealthy in the first place. If you will bask in the love of the journey, then the work He will do will be lasting, lifelong, never to have to be revisited again.

Oh, how many strongholds have I revisited in my life simply because in my impatience I did not allow Him to complete the work that needed to be done. Don't be afraid to allow God to go deep. ***Psalm 139:23-24***. ***Search me O God, and know my heart. Try me and know my anxieties: and see if there is any wicked way in me, and lead me into the way everlasting.***

Allow God to do this during this twelve weeks. Let Him do your makeover! The everlasting makeover!

The Bible talks about the true ultimate makeover. It is 2 Corinthians 5:17. If anyone be in Christ he is a new creation, old things are passed away, behold all things become new.

This session we will discuss how to approach God:

Session Notes...

Write 1 John 5:14-15...

# *God is Love . . . . Journal Pages*

Now this is the confidence-

1 John 5:14-15.

*Psalm 19 (New International Version)*

*Psalm 19*
*For the director of music. A psalm of David.*

*[1] The heavens declare the glory of God;*
*the skies proclaim the work of his hands.*
*[2] Day after day they pour forth speech;*
*night after night they display knowledge.*
*[3] There is no speech or language*
*where their voice is not heard.*
*[4] Their voice goes out into all the earth,*
*their words to the ends of the world.*
*In the heavens he has pitched a tent for the sun,*
*[5] which is like a bridegroom coming forth from his pavilion,*
*like a champion rejoicing to run his course.*
*[6] It rises at one end of the heavens*
*and makes its circuit to the other;*
*nothing is hidden from its heat.*
*[7] The law of the LORD is perfect,*
*reviving the soul.*
*The statutes of the LORD are trustworthy,*
*making wise the simple.*
*[8] The precepts of the LORD are right,*
*giving joy to the heart.*
*The commands of the LORD are radiant,*
*giving light to the eyes.*
*[9] The fear of the LORD is pure,*
*enduring forever.*
*The ordinances of the LORD are sure*
*and altogether righteous.*
*[10] They are more precious than gold,*
*than much pure gold;*
*they are sweeter than honey,*
*than honey from the comb.*
*[11] By them is your servant warned;*
*in keeping them there is great reward.*
*[12] Who can discern his errors?*
*Forgive my hidden faults.*

*13 Keep your servant also from willful sins;*
*may they not rule over me.*
*Then will I be blameless,*
*innocent of great transgression.*
*14 May the words of my mouth and the meditation of my heart*
*be pleasing in your sight,*
*O LORD, my Rock and my Redeemer.*

# Session Seven. We Belong to God.

***Memory Scripture: Romans 8:6-17 The Spirit Himself bears witness with our spirit that we are children of God, and if children, then heirs of God and joint heirs with Christ, if we indeed suffer with Him, that we may also be glorified together.***

When my daughter, Kim, was a little girl, she used to sing a song about being adopted. I remember some of the chorus, it was, "I am adopted, I'm a special kid you see, there's room in His big kingdom for a little kid like me," and it goes on to talk about how God has adopted us and we have become part of His family. In Romans, we are assured that at the moment we receive Jesus, we *are* adopted by God and become His child. We can call Him "Father." From then on, we are part of the family of God...joint heirs with Jesus Christ. There is nothing that can take that away. This is definitely an adoption that is final! Praise God!

When we receive that wonderful, eternal gift of salvation, that is not the end, it is only the beginning! While we are here, our purpose is to serve and worship Him. He has paid the price for our sins, we are forgiven. It is so wonderful to call Him, "Abba Father."

We are no longer to live according to the flesh, but by the Spirit, which now lives inside of us. Let's start eating and exercising like we are children of God. We need much energy and strength to serve Him and be our best for Him. ***Romans 8:1*** tells us...***Therefore, there is now no condemnation for those who are in Christ Jesus.*** We have been set free from the law by Christ and what He did for us. Have you accepted full freedom from Christ? Even though God is not condemning us, we continue to condemn ourselves. <u>It is so hard for some of us to allow ourselves to be completely free.</u> We continue to struggle with feelings of unworthiness and self loathing. This is not how God wants us to live. When we come to Christ, at that moment when He forgives our sins, all is forgiven. The past, present and future sins are included in that. It is not God that is causing us to live less than an abundant life. It is our own condemnation of ourselves that holds us back from true freedom in Christ. We simply have a hard time accepting the gift of salvation. When we begin to walk in the Spirit as it talks about in Romans, then all of our desires will change. We will truly be like, look like and act like children of God. During this session, we will discuss being children of God and living according to the Spirit.

Session Notes…

Write Romans 8:16-17…

# *Journal Pages*

The Spirit

-Romans 8:16-17.

## *Psalm 145*

*A psalm of praise. Of David.*
*1 I will exalt you, my God the King;*
*I will praise your name for ever and ever.*
*2 Every day I will praise you*
*and extol your name for ever and ever.*
*3 Great is the LORD and most worthy of praise;*
*his greatness no one can fathom.*
*4 One generation will commend your works to another;*
*they will tell of your mighty acts.*
*5 They will speak of the glorious splendor of your majesty,*
*and I will meditate on your wonderful works.*
*6 They will tell of the power of your awesome works,*
*and I will proclaim your great deeds.*
*7 They will celebrate your abundant goodness*
*and joyfully sing of your righteousness.*
*8 The LORD is gracious and compassionate,*
*slow to anger and rich in love.*
*9 The LORD is good to all;*
*he has compassion on all he has made.*
*10 All you have made will praise you, O LORD;*
*your saints will extol you.*
*11 They will tell of the glory of your kingdom*
*and speak of your might,*
*12 so that all men may know of your mighty acts*
*and the glorious splendor of your kingdom.*
*13 Your kingdom is an everlasting kingdom,*
*and your dominion endures through all generations.*
*The LORD is faithful to all his promises*
*and loving toward all he has made.*
*14 The LORD upholds all those who fall*
*and lifts up all who are bowed down.*
*15 The eyes of all look to you,*
*and you give them their food at the proper time.*
*16 You open your hand*
*and satisfy the desires of every living thing.*
*17 The LORD is righteous in all his ways*
*and loving toward all he has made.*

*18 The LORD is near to all who call on him,*
*to all who call on him in truth.*
*19 He fulfills the desires of those who fear him;*
*he hears their cry and saves them.*
*20 The LORD watches over all who love him,*
*but all the wicked he will destroy.*
*21 My mouth will speak in praise of the LORD.*
*Let every creature praise his holy name*
*for ever and ever.*

# Session Eight. Casting our Cares/Stress Reduction.

***Memory Scripture: 1 Peter 5:6-7 Therefore humble yourselves under the mighty hand of God, that He may exalt you in due time. Cast all of your cares upon Him for He cares for you.***

I have lived long enough now to realize what a blessed invitation that is when He tells me to cast all of my cares upon Him! What a Savior! What a relief! Thank You, Lord, that I do not have to handle all of this myself, because there is no way that I can do it.

When I think of the word *cast*, I cannot help but think of my childhood and spending many days with my Daddy on a lake bank. He was a champion fisherman, and knew just about everything there was to know about the sport of fishing. One of the first things he taught me to do was to cast a line. There is definitely an art to it. There is no holding back; you have to get everything in position and just at the right time you have to let go and cast the line over the water. I think of this when I think of casting my cares upon God. It is truly a relief and blessing to know that God is in control and we are not. Of course, those rods do have reels on them. Sometimes I cast it to Him and then I reel it back. That is not good. I'm sure that you have probably done the same thing, but again, with God's help, we will learn to trust Him and let go of the things that are hindering our service to Him. When we truly let go and cast our burdens far out to Him—no reeling back—then, the He will take care of things for us.

Don't forget the last part of the verse. Why is He willing to shoulder our burdens? Because He cares for us, He loves us, He is Sovereign, He knows what is best for us, He is in control, and He has a plan for us and our families. He will meet our every need. He is God!

Casting our cares upon God is a vital part of this program because of the stress reduction. Stress can affect our health in so many negative ways. Many people are stress eaters. When life drops stressful situations into our laps, we tend to eat too much, eat too little, and forget to hydrate, forget about exercise, or exercise too much, and so on. In other words, our discipline goes out the window. There are many life situations that are very devastating and many times life cannot go on as usual. All of us have experienced life interruptions. Ask God to help you use the circle of health when these life interruptions happen to you.

Maybe you are experiencing:

- Illness in your family
- Death of loved one
- Separation or divorce
- Marital problems
- Prodigal child
- Becoming caretaker for elderly parent or parents
- Job change or loss
- Relationship problems
- Health problems
- Financial problems
- Having to relocate
- Physical changes

This list could go on and on: you can probably make your own list. All of these have happened to at least one person I know in the last year. Each one of them is very difficult to deal with and causes tremendous stress.

Trusting God and knowing that He is with us is even more precious during the hard times. I am always needy and in need of God, more every day, but when these things occur, it makes me even more aware of my need for Him. (***2 Thessalonians 2:16-17) May our Lord Jesus Christ himself and God our Father, who loved us and by his grace gave us*** eternal encouragement ***and good hope encourage your hearts and strengthen you in every good deed and word.*** God is our greatest encourager. He is forever looking after us and wanting the best for us. When these trials come to us, the enemy would love for us to turn away from God. He knows that when we do that, then he has us right where he wants us. Don't do it! Cry out to God, lean on Him, bask in His eternal encouragement! He will bring you through whatever it is that you are going through.

As our Father is encouraging us, let's discuss ways to encourage each other. Will you learn to cast today?

Session Notes...

Write 1 Peter 5:6-7...

# *Journal Pages*

Write 1 Peter 5:6-7

# *Journal Pages..*

## *Psalm 121*

***A song for pilgrims ascending to Jerusalem.***

*1 I look up to the mountains—*
*does my help come from there?*
*2 My help comes from the Lord,*
*who made heaven and earth!*
*3 He will not let you stumble;*
*the one who watches over you will not slumber.*
*4 Indeed, he who watches over Israel*
*never slumbers or sleeps.*
*5 The Lord himself watches over you!*
*The Lord stands beside you as your protective shade.*
*6 The sun will not harm you by day,*
*nor the moon at night.*
*7 The Lord keeps you from all harm*
*and watches over your life.*
*8 The Lord keeps watch over you as you come and go,*
*both now and forever.*

# Session Nine. Don't Worry-Be Healthy Stress Reduction.

***Memory Scripture: Philippians 4:4-7 Rejoice in the Lord always, again I say Rejoice! Let your gentleness be known to all men, the Lord is at hand. Be anxious for nothing, but in everything by prayer and supplication, with thanksgiving, let your requests be made known to God, and the peace of God which surpasses all understanding, will guard your hearts and minds through Christ Jesus.***

How much have you changed or gained in your life by worrying? How much of your thought life is spent in worry or with thoughts that are not in line with our scripture verse? God does not want us to waste time and energy worrying. This may sound harsh but I am talking to myself too… worrying is a sin! It is not the way God meant for us to exist, in a constant state of panic and worry, wringing our hands about things that have happened, might happen, and might not happen…and so on and so on. I believe the enemy loves to get us in a state of panic and worry. I have seen it happen in my own family.

***In Matthew 6:25 it says "Therefore I tell you, do not worry about your life, what you will eat or drink; or about your body, what you will wear. Is not life more important than food and the body more important than clothes?"***

There are so many more times God's word speaks against worrying. It tells us not to worry about tomorrow.

When we are constantly worrying about something, it is because we are still trying to take part of the control. Somehow, we still think that we can fix things.

When we are in the habit of worrying, we can be taking in many more calories than we realize. Are you the stress eater we talked about last week? Have you ever turned to food to satisfy a need? At times when we are under pressure from those family problems, economic situations, relationship issues and other things, we can let our food intake get out of control. It is not only the amount of food that gets out of control; it is also *what* we eat. Have you ever noticed when you are stressed out or worried about something, you don't usually go for a stalk of celery or a carrot? No, it tends to be a brownie, ice cream, cake, or donut…on and on…

When we finally release control of our lives to God, then the worry stops and the peace begins. By turning to Him in prayer, minute by minute, the anxiety leaves us and His peace replaces it. The knowledge that God is in control gives us that blessed peace of mind that ends all worry.

Worry is a habit. It has to be broken just like any other bad habit or stronghold. Remember...***anything that causes us...*** you know the rest. Whenever you start to worry or have anxious thoughts, immediately go to God in prayer. Do it aloud if you can. Rejoice in the Lord. Sing out loud to Him. Call on the name of Jesus. Say the name of Jesus out loud. Remember, there is power, strength, healing, peace, and so much more in the name of Jesus. Let this become the new habit, replacing the old habit of worry and anxiety.

I come from a long line of worriers! Some of the most influential ladies in my life were constantly living in the world of 'what if.' I love all of them, but years ago I had to break free from living under the weight of what could happen. I choose to believe that God has my best interest at heart. If I even start to return to old ways, I remind myself with God's word that He is in control and is looking out for me and my family. His plans are much better than ours and we are in His hands.( ***Isaiah 40:11) He tends his flock like a shepherd. He gathers the lambs in his arms and carries them close to His heart. He gently leads those that have young.*** To this day, there are many times when I have to speak to God aloud saying, "You are in control and I am not!" I repeat it over and over. This battles the enemy's attack until he gives up and leaves me alone. Living with worry is bondage. It can keep us from doing many of the things we could and should be doing.

Like with all of the habits we are changing on this program, don't wait! Let's start right now...and now is when the peace will begin!

Session Notes... Use this session to identify if you may be a stress eater. Make a plan of action to use the next time you are tempted to satisfy a need with food.

______________________________________________

______________________________________________

______________________________________________

______________________________________________

______________________________________________

______________________________________________

Write Philippians 4:4-7.

# *Journal Pages*

*Philippians 4:4-7.*

# *Journal Pages . . . Relaxation . . .*

*Psalm 30 (New International Version)*

*[1] I will exalt you, O LORD,*
*for you lifted me out of the depths*
*and did not let my enemies gloat over me.*
*[2] O LORD my God, I called to you for help*
*and you healed me.*
*[3] O LORD, you brought me up from the grave ;*
*you spared me from going down into the pit.*
*[4] Sing to the LORD, you saints of his;*
*praise his holy name.*
*[5] For his anger lasts only a moment,*
*but his favor lasts a lifetime;*
*weeping may remain for a night,*
*but rejoicing comes in the morning.*
*[6] When I felt secure, I said,*
*"I will never be shaken."*
*[7] O LORD, when you favored me,*
*you made my mountain stand firm;*
*but when you hid your face,*
*I was dismayed.*

*[8] To you, O LORD, I called;*
*to the Lord I cried for mercy:*
*[9] "What gain is there in my destruction,*
*in my going down into the pit?*
*Will the dust praise you?*
*Will it proclaim your faithfulness?*
*[10] Hear, O LORD, and be merciful to me;*
*O LORD, be my help."*
*[11] You turned my wailing into dancing;*
*you removed my sackcloth and clothed me with joy,*
*[12] that my heart may sing to you and not be silent.*
*O LORD my God, I will give you thanks forever.*

# Session Ten. Choose the Good Part! Stress Reduction.

***Memory Scripture: Luke 10:42 But one thing is needed and Mary has chosen the good part, which will not be taken away from her.***

***Read Luke 10:38-42.***

When thinking about how to reduce stress in our lives, we can't very well ignore the story of Martha and Mary. Poor Martha was running herself ragged trying to be an excellent hostess, and look at the reaction from Jesus. Look at verse 40. ***(Luke 10:40a) But Martha was distracted by all the preparations that had to be made.*** Do you think that if Jesus came to your house today, you would be distracted? Would any meal preparation or duties that had to be done take priority over sitting at His feet?

But…He is at our house today. He is waiting to spend time with us. He wants our undivided attention, where we focus on nothing but Him. His Word is lying there waiting to be read. He has something new to show us each and every day. But, like Martha, we are distracted. We are busy, we are serving, we are running households, we are parenting, we are working jobs…we are simply too busy to sit at His feet.

We, like Martha, are killing ourselves for the temporal things and missing out on the good part! He referred to it as the good part. The eternal, that which cannot be taken away! That is what Mary chose. I don't want to miss the good part. Do you?

So…somebody's got to do the Martha thing!

I read something one time that has stuck with me for many years. It simply said, "Every time you say NO, it opens a door for someone else to say YES."

Stress Reduction: Pray and ask God to guide you in daily living to be more like Mary. What do you need to remove from your life that could simplify your life and the life of your family? Over scheduling is a great attack on family life. I have seen it in my own family. As a part of this program, seek God's will to develop a schedule that is pleasing to Him. Make time for all components of the circle of health, and especially for the component of stress reduction. Consider your alone time at Jesus' feet to be a life priority. We all want to experience the good part!

Discussion... how to simplify our lives...

Session Notes...

Write...Luke 10: 42.

# *Journal Pages*

*CHOOSE THE GOOD PART*

*Luke 10:42.*

# Journal Pages.. Eating triggers . . .

*These things I have spoken to you, that in Me you may have peace. In the world, you will have tribulation; be of good cheer, I have overcome the world. John 16:33*

*From the Hymn: Jesus the Very Thought of Thee*

*<u>Jesus the Very Thought of Thee</u>*

*Jesus, the very thought of Thee with sweetness fills my breast,*
*But sweeter far Thy face to see and in Thy presence rest.*

*No voice can sing, no heart can frame, nor can the memory find,*
*A sweeter sound than Thy blest name, O Savior of mankind.*

*O hope of every contrite heart, O joy of all the meek,*
*To those who fall, how kind Thou art, How good to those who seek.*

*Jesus, our only joy be Thou, As Thou our prize wilt be,*
*Jesus be Thou our glory now, and through eternity.*

*To Sit at the Feet of Jesus*

# Session Eleven. Come Unto Jesus.

The Ultimate Stress Reduction

***Memory Scripture: Matthew 11:28-30 Come unto me all you who labor and are heavy laden, and I will give you rest. Take my yoke upon you and learn from me, for I am gentle and lowly in heart and you will find rest for your souls. For my yoke is easy and my burden is light.***

Are you carrying a heavy burden? Are you heavy with panic, anxiety or worry? Are you crippled by fear? Do you constantly labor and get no rest?

Yes, our bodies need sufficient rest…but Jesus is offering rest for our souls! What a rest that is! That is the ultimate, peace of mind, Peace of God rest!

There was a time in my life that I was not sure about the state of my salvation. I had walked the aisle as a very young child and had joined the church and been baptized. Now, I have no doubt whatsoever that God can and does save young children of all ages. But, for me, later on in my young adult life, I was heavy laden with doubts. I carried this burden with me everywhere. I simply wasn't sure. My soul was not at rest.

A series of events happened in my life in my early 30s that really made me begin to question my salvation. One was the death of my Grandmother and then the death of my Father. As hard as I tried, I had no surety that I would see them again in Heaven. I tried to talk with people and get some help with this, but they would usually just assure me that I was OK and tell me that everyone has doubts and that it was normal. I knew down deep inside that what I was feeling was not normal and that I was not supposed to be tormented with these doubts. This was true bondage, especially for a good little Baptist girl, and now grown up lady with children.

This went on and on and My husband Mike and I would even talk about it from time to time. Then I would go to church and play the piano like everything was great. It wasn't!

The one thing that kept coming to my mind when people would assure me that it was the enemy attacking me was: why would the enemy attack me so and cause me to constantly doubt my salvation? If I thought I was saved and I was not, it seemed to me like that would be perfect for him. Why wouldn't he just leave me alone?

On a Sunday morning during a revival, the visiting pastor preached on the story of the wheat and the tares. I knew immediately he was talking about me. The Holy Spirit told me that now was the time to get this straight. I knew that this was the day that I would talk to someone and ask for help until I got it. When he gave the invitation, many people came forward, and I wanted to come also…I honestly felt like God was speaking to me and allowing me to have this last chance to get this right. Complication!! I was playing the invitation and people were coming! Now if any of you are church musicians, you know that one of our goals in life is to not create a distraction during the invitation. I really couldn't believe that no one out there could hear the beating of my heart. I thought it would surely beat out of my chest. So…the invitation came and went…but my heart pounded on and I knew that I would not go home that day until I had talked with someone. As soon as the service was over, I approached a fellow musician who was also a decision time counselor. I shared my story with him and we prayed the prayer of salvation. I did not want to doubt anything that had happened when I was a child, I simply wanted to get right with God and be sure that I was saved. That is what happened that day. I told God exactly how I felt; I confessed my sin and told Him I needed Him. God saved me! I asked Jesus to come into my heart and I also prayed for the doubts to leave. They did!

Was I embarrassed to tell anyone? No! Because I had been serving at the church? No! How was I going to tell it or explain it? I could not wait to tell it! I can honestly say that whatever pride I might have had was completely gone at this time. There is no pride that feels better than being obedient to God! Anyway, I wanted to tell everyone, in case any one I knew was going through the same thing!

Mike had to work that day, but as soon as he arrived home that afternoon, I told him what had happened. I also told him that he didn't have to doubt, that he too could know for sure. I told him this because we had been having conversations about this and I wanted him to be sure also. So, that night at church, he went forward and prayed. We were both baptized at Harp's Crossing Church. ***James 1: 6-8. But when he asks, he must believe and not doubt, because he who doubts is like a wave of the sea, blown and tossed by the wind. That man should not think he will receive anything from the Lord; he is a double-minded man, unstable in all he does.*** This was me before! No peace, easily tossed!

I want to be totally honest. I still do not know what happened to me that day as a child…just like many people I know that have been through this or a similar experience, I really can't remember much about my experience as a young child. The one thing God has made clear to me is that whether I was or was not saved as a child, I was obedient to Him that Sunday at Harp's Crossing. There is no better feeling in the world than being sure of your salvation! Praise the Lord! He is so good!

There is no heavier burden than not knowing if you are right with God. There can be no greater cause of stress. I don't want anyone reading this to go through the years that I had to go through by putting this off. I spoke with a friend recently who told me that she prays the prayer every time the invitation is given just in case. There is no "Just in case" ya'll! God wants us to be sure about our eternal life!

Do you know Jesus? Are you sure about your salvation? Are you headed for Heaven? He invites each of us to come to Him. He wants to take away this heavy burden. He wants to save us from our sins. He is ready and waiting to forgive and save you.

All you have to do is realize and acknowledge that you are a sinner and are not able to save yourself. Believe that Jesus Christ is the Son of God, confess your sins to God and ask Him to come into your heart and save you.

He will do it. There is nothing else we have to do to be saved. We could never be good enough to be right with God. Only through Jesus Christ! If you have prayed the prayer, you can be sure that you are saved and you should tell someone about this wonderful thing that has happened to you!

Maybe you have been saved, but have not been living as you know God would have you to. Or maybe you have simply not been growing in the Lord. Again, you can come to Him right now and turn your life over to Him completely. He is ready to move forward. He is ready and waiting to forgive sin. He is ready to carry that burden for you and give you peace. Pray and recommit your life to God. He is only a prayer away.

The months after I asked Jesus into my heart and was obedient to God were the months when I lost the weight. Please choose freedom! Freedom is Jesus Christ!

# Journal Pages

*Write...Matthew 11:28-30*

*Psalm 103 (New American Standard Bible)*

***Praise for the LORD'S Mercies.***
***A Psalm of David.***

***1Bless the LORD, O my soul,***
***And all that is within me, bless His holy name.***
***2Bless the LORD, O my soul,***
***And forget none of His benefits;***
***3Who pardons all your iniquities,***
***Who heals all your diseases;***
***4Who redeems your life from the pit,***
***Who crowns you with lovingkindness and compassion;***
***5Who satisfies your years with good things,***
***So that your youth is renewed like the eagle.***
***6The LORD performs righteous deeds***
***And judgments for all who are oppressed.***
***7He made known His ways to Moses,***
***His acts to the sons of Israel.***
***8The LORD is compassionate and gracious,***
***Slow to anger and abounding in lovingkindness.***
***9He will not always strive with us,***
***Nor will He keep His anger forever.***
***10He has not dealt with us according to our sins,***
***Nor rewarded us according to our iniquities.***
***11For as high as the heavens are above the earth,***
***So great is His lovingkindness toward those who fear Him.***
***12As far as the east is from the west,***
***So far has He removed our transgressions from us.***
***13Just as a father has compassion on his children,***
***So the LORD has compassion on those who fear Him.***
***14For He Himself knows our frame;***
***He is mindful that we are but dust.***
***15As for man, his days are like grass;***
***As a flower of the field, so he flourishes.***
***16When the wind has passed over it, it is no more,***
***And its place acknowledges it no longer.***
***17But the lovingkindness of the LORD is from***

*everlasting to everlasting on those who fear Him,*
*And His righteousness to children's children,*
18 *To those who keep His covenant*
*And remember His precepts to do them.*
19 *The LORD has established His throne in the heavens,*
*And His sovereignty rules over all.*
20 *Bless the LORD, you His angels,*
*Mighty in strength, who perform His word,*
*Obeying the voice of His word!*
21 *Bless the LORD, all you His hosts,*
*You who serve Him, doing His will.*
22 *Bless the LORD, all you works of His,*
*In all places of His dominion;*
*Bless the LORD, O my soul!*

# Session Twelve. Be Free.

Fit for His Service

***Memory Scripture: John 10:10 The thief does not come except to steal and kill and destroy. I have come that they may have life and that they may have it more abundantly.***

Jesus came to take us from death to life, from darkness into light. He is that light. We belong to Him. We are His servants. He not only wants us to have life, but to have abundant life. He meant for us to live life serving Him to the fullest. ***A life of intensity.***

The enemy wants us sick, tired, beaten down, unhappy, unhealthy, overweight, doubtful, ashamed, stressed out, and so on and so on…But God is greater and the victory has already been won. He has died to give us a life of freedom and he does not want us to go back into captivity.

I am sure you will agree with me when I say that I do not believe that there are any random words in the Bible. God's Word is so perfect and precise. Jesus said He came, lived, died on the cross and lives again so we can have abundant life! There is one thing even greater than all of those I just listed and that is, He lives in our hearts! He did not say He came so we could have a mediocre, half-way, ordinary life. <u>He said abundant!</u> That is the way I believe He wants us to live.

Jesus has come to set the captives free! (I***saiah 61:1) The Spirit of the Lord GOD is upon me; because the LORD hath anointed me to preach good tidings unto the meek; he hath sent me to bind up the brokenhearted, to*** <u>proclaim liberty to the captives</u>***, and the*** <u>opening of the prison to them that are bound.</u> I pray that the last twelve weeks has opened up your prison doors and set you free!

He wants us free from unhealthy eating, from a sedentary lifestyle, from dehydration, from stress and anxiety…from anything that hinders our service and walk with Him.

You have accomplished twelve weeks on a new course, a new way of eating, living, moving, and thinking. I ask God to help you continue on this course you are on, to a better, healthier way of life. I pray that you and your family have benefited and will continue to grow healthy as you stay on the program. May we encourage each other to continue this lifestyle and commit to pray for each other daily.

This session will be a discussion on the plans God has for our service to Him. Let's begin a life of intensity!

Session notes…

______________________________________________
______________________________________________
______________________________________________
______________________________________________
______________________________________________
______________________________________________

Write John 10:10…

______________________________________________
______________________________________________

# *Journal Pages*

*Be Free…Be Free!*

*Greater is He that is in me..Greater is He that is in me…Greater is He that is in me than he that is in the world!*

*Write…John 10:10*

# *Journal Pages*

*Make a joyful noise unto the Lord, all you lands!*
*Serve the Lord with gladness!*
*Come before His presence with singing.*
*Know that the Lord, He is God.*
*It is He who has made us and not we ourselves.*
*We are His people and the sheep of His pasture.*
*Enter into His gates with thanksgiving, and into His courts with praise!*
*Be thankful to Him and Bless His Name!*
*For the Lord is good!*
*His mercy is everlasting*
*And*
*His truth endures to all generations.*
*Psalm 100*

LaVergne, TN USA
04 November 2010
203542LV00003B/6/P

9 781615 072255